Forward

Dentistry has changed quite a bit since I got started forty years ago. Procedures are more complicated, equipment is more advanced and patients are different too. They're more educated and inquisitive. Our consumer no longer picks the practice closest to their home or office. They want and demand more from us. The world has changed – the game has changed.

As small business owners, we wear a lot of hats. And other than being the best dentist in your zipcode, being a great marketer is also incredibly important. Think about it - until a stranger becomes a patient, they will never know what a great clinician you are. So, even though you're at the top of your game, no one knows it until you get them in the door. Consider your favorite restaurant. You go there for the food (what's inside), but great ones invest in the entire experience. They invest in how the business looks from the outside, the parking lot, the signage, the service and the staff so they can get you to come inside and spend money. A solid brand is just the beginning of the relationship.

I have read many books on marketing a dental practice. This is the very first book on what I feel is the very first critical step in getting the marketing right - BRANDING your practice. This book shows the importance of consumer branding and captures the essence of building a brand for YOUR practice. It's presented in an easy to read, step-by-step process that leads you to DISCOVERING YOUR OWN BRAND.

I'm confident that every dentist will find something in this book they can put into practice immediately to build their personal and practice brand.

Dr. Joe Blaes

BRANDING IN PRACTICE

The little black book of branding secrets that is an absolute necessity to a dentist's success

By

Matthew Petchel

& Joanne Lee

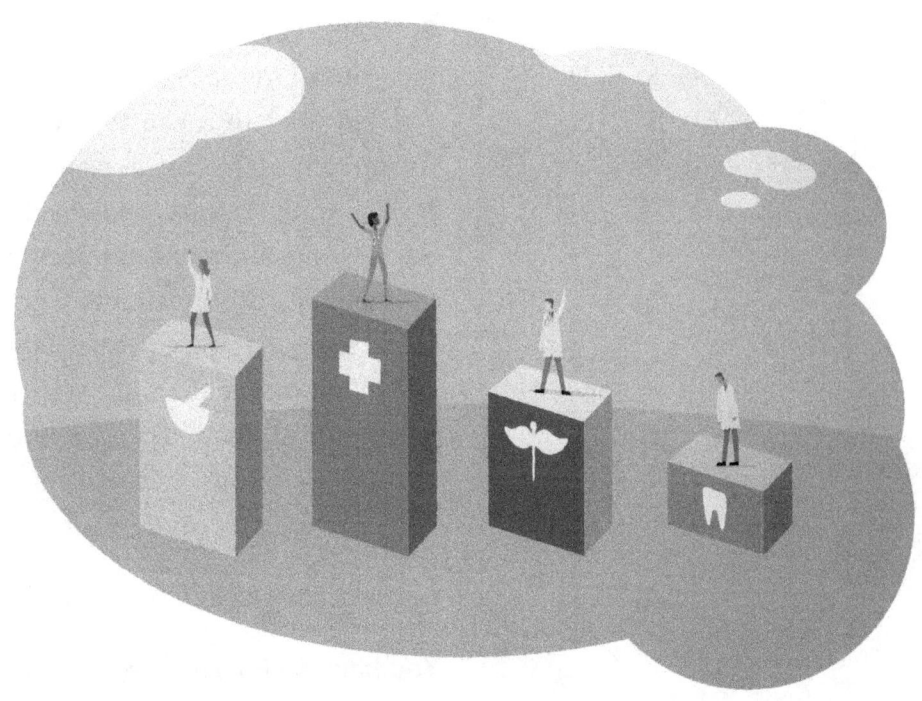

People don't trust you

...as much as they trust doctors, nurses, pharmacists and engineers.

Here's how you rate when respondents were asked if these people were trustworthy.

	% Very high/ High
Nurses	85
Pharmacists	75
Medical doctors	70
Engineers	70
Dentists	62
Police officers	58
College teachers	53
Clergy	52
Psychiatrists	41
Chiropractors	38
Bankers	28
Journalists	24
Business executives	21
State governors	20
Lawyers	19
Insurance salespeople	15
Senators	14
HMO Managers	12
Stockbrokers	11
Advertising practitioners	11
Members of Congress	10
Car salespeople	8

Gallup, Nov. 26-29, 2012

But wait...you are a trust-worthy individual. You pay your taxes. You tell the truth. You turn your phone off while the airplane is taxiing on the tarmac. So, why do doctors, nurses, and pharmacists (all healthcare professionals) get more love and respect than you do? What makes them different? What makes them special? The answer is both simple and complicated.

Dentists have an image problem.

You have an image problem. And branding could be the cure.

In this little book of secrets, we're going to show you how to fix this. And fortunately for you, many dentists will never take the initiative and read this, so you will survive and thrive while many of your colleagues will just get by.

Let's start by first explaining what a brand is.

http://www.gallup.com/poll/159035/congress-retains-low-honesty-rating.asp

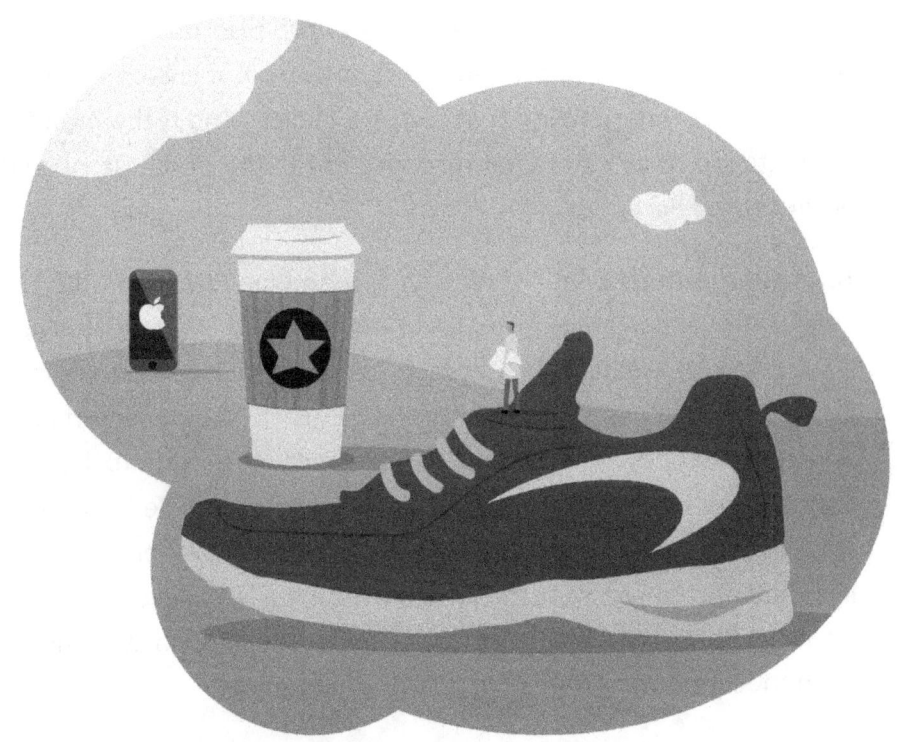

What Is A Brand?

Brands are all around us. They're in our hands, they're on our feet, in our coffee cups, speaking to us on TV, parked in our driveways and waiting to serve us. We all know they exist, but why do they exist? And how do they become what they are? It's not by accident. A brand is incredibly deliberate and it's why we believe those sneakers will make us better athletes, why that cup of coffee makes us feel happy and why that car makes us feel successful or secure. It's why we buy these things. It's why we buy things again and again. And it's why you, as a dental professional, should consider becoming a brand of your own.

First things first...let's define the term 'brand'. It's not easy to do, as it's one of the most intangible and misconstrued terms around.

Simply defined, a brand is the personal promise of a product or service that elicits an emotional response from a customer. It's a subconscious inner feeling that forces a choice. And if the brand is doing its job, that emotional response elicits the purchase of that product or service.

To give an example, let's start with a brand leader...Nike. It's the quintessential consumer product brand that empowers us to 'Just Do It'. And by wearing that swoosh, we truly believe that we can. Everything Nike says, does and shows us in their marketing is related to empowerment and performance. We start to believe that LeBron's jump-shot, Rory's drive are all propelled, in some way, by that Nike logo that they wear. We want to perform just like they do. So we want the swoosh. And we're willing to spend a lot more for a pair of sneakers to get it even though we'll never even touch the rim. That's the power of branding.

To give another example, Apple is the model consumer product brand that empowers us to 'Think Differently'. And by using an iMac, iPhone, iPad or Apple Watch, we truly believe that we can work faster, smarter and more creatively. Everything Apple says, does and shows us in their marketing is related to empowerment and performance. We start to believe that piece of technology can make a difference in our lives. It can make us better, faster, smarter. So we want the i-whatever. And we're willing to spend a lot more for it. That's the power of branding.

When we first think of brands, we usually think of products — phones, sneakers, cars, toothpastes, cereals, etc. But branding touches almost anything that needs to be seen or sold. Sure, Starbucks is selling the product of coffee, but their brand isn't just about the coffee. Their brand is about the experience...or the "third place", as they call it. They wanted to be the place that isn't home or work, where you go to relax and enjoy. They provided comfy couches, cool music and a familiar environment. They called their coffee pourers 'baristas', paid them well and gave them health benefits so they'd be able to hire the best customer servers. They created a coffee menu that's longer than most diner menus, but that caters to every customer's individual tastes. The whole experience tells the customer he or she is special. And who wouldn't want to spend time (and money) at a third place like that?

People themselves have become brands. Athletes are brands and, in the competitive world of sponsorships, their carefully crafted image can be the difference between having The Four Seasons as a sponsor or Super 8. Celebrities are 'celebrated' and adored because they represent an image and promise to their fans. Donald Trump is a proven capitalist, but he is also a constructed brand, promising the dream of material success. Everything he does and says paints that dream.

Even medical professionals have learned to brand themselves. Just look at Dr. Oz or Dr. Phil. They are common household brand names now. Dr. Mehmet Oz, an acclaimed cardiothoracic surgeon became a guest expert on Oprah and then extended his brand to carry his own successful daytime show. His brand promises to advocate healthy living. He makes his brand compelling by making the human body fascinating, yet relatable, and giving medical advice in a motivating way. He lives his brand by eating healthy and always appearing lean, energetic, confident, and...healthy. He evangelizes his brand across the world, through his show, his books, XM/Sirius radio and the internet.

For service professionals to be truly successful, they need to embody the promise of their brand. Dentists don't need to be TV stars, but they should represent an image that appeals to their audience and supports the brand of their practice.

It's branding personified...and it's how you will take your business to the next level.

Think of it this way. A potential patient has no 'real' experience with what a great clinician you are since they've never met you. But your brand does a lot of the talking for you BEFORE they even meet you. **Branding helps get them in the door.**

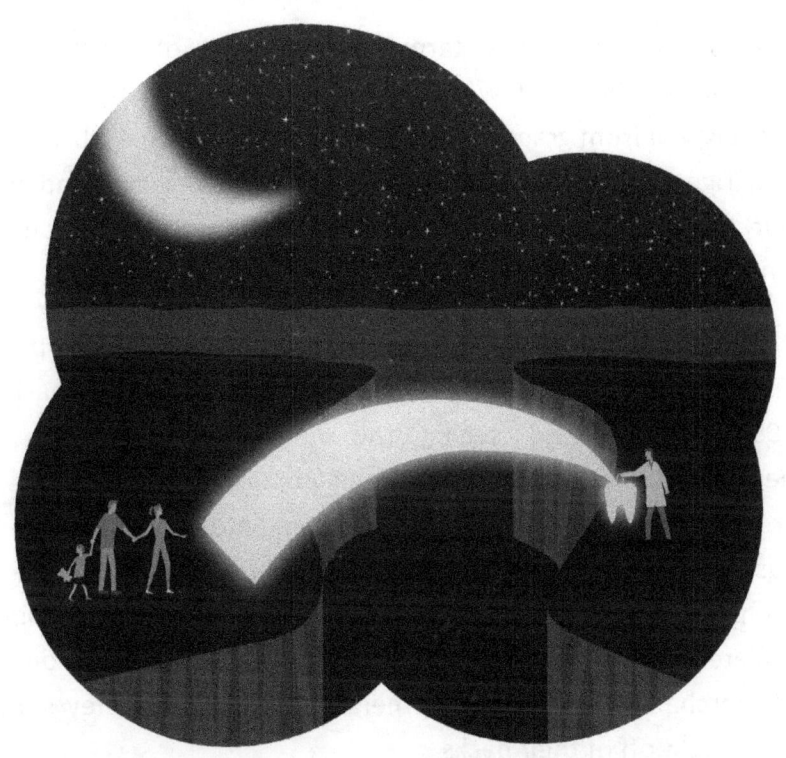

In Brands We Trust

The exact emotional response we feel when we experience (buy, wear, drink, eat, drive, watch, etc.) a brand is different based on the product or service that we're experiencing. However, the underlying emotion that is common to all successful brands is trust. We trust that when we leave Starbucks, we will be energized and ready to take on the day. We trust that we'll get service with a smile and that the 1/2-caf, double shot, Venti, 2-pump vanilla, non-fat, extra-hot, latte will be our idyllic cup of coffee. If consumers trust a brand, they'll engage with it and purchase it – usually without giving it much thought.

The converse, of course, is true as well. If consumers don't trust a brand, they'll defect. Although Nike is still one of the strongest brands on earth, they tarnished the trust of many of their customers when a few of their sponsored athletes and 'role-models' fell from grace. We trusted Nike because we trusted Lance and Tiger. And Nike now has to work hard to regain and rebuild our trust – with new sponsorships, more powerful promotion, sincere advertising...and even greater products.

The one element we can't always (or ever) trust is the competition. They're continually circling and we need to watch our backs. In 1996, Nike missed seeing the need/opportunity for 'high-performance under shirts'. Along comes Under Armour. They created a category (that it still dominates) and wooed Nike customers with products that compete with everything Nike sells. From t-shirts, to running shoes, to footballs to everything an athlete would wear. In 2013, Under Armour sold $2.3 Billion worth of merchandise to Nike customers. You might say they stole the shirts right off of their backs.

Competition is everywhere. Yours might be the dentist down the street. He or she is actively looking for those opportunities that you've missed. But it's just as likely to be the things your potential patients choose to buy with their disposable income...like jewelry, handbags, golf clubs, flat screen TVs, or anything else that costs around $1,000. It's up to you to make your solutions for oral health and beautiful teeth the more attractive, and better, purchasing choice.

Emotions... trust... courting... engagement... They all seem like characteristics of a relationship. And that is exactly what a brand establishes with its customer. It's a relationship that the brand owner hopes will last a lifetime. And, as we all know, relationships require hard work and dedication.

Think of the car you drive. As Americans, our cars are one of our most treasured relationships. We take a lot of time researching and test driving them. We work hard to pay for them. We wash them and take them in for check-ups. Some of us even give our cars names. But usually the first thing that pops into our minds when we think of our cars is the brand. Volvo, Mercedes, Ford, BMW, Volkswagen, Mini, etc. The list of brands goes on and on. And each brand establishes a very deliberate relationship with its driver.

Take Toyota, for example. If you drive a Toyota, you probably value reliability. But so do most drivers. What you REALLY want out of your relationship with your car is to be environmentally (and financially) responsible. So you buy a Prius. With the advent of the Prius in 1997, Toyota was the first to mass-market a hybrid car. They dropped anchor in the sustainability space and are still top-of-mind for most consumers when we think of environmentally-friendly cars. They've capitalized on the image over the years and are very deliberate in communicating their mission, for example:

Environmental Responsibility

From the development of sustainable vehicles and making manufacturing plants sustainable to vehicle recycling, 'eco-driving' educational programs and reforestation, Toyota is actively engaged in a wide variety of programs to improve the environment.

- Toyota Global Website

Most of Toyota's initiatives are related to that global responsibility. Most everything they communicate to their customers is trying to appeal to the emotions related to responsibility - to make them trust the car and the brand. BMW wants the driver who values sport and luxury. Volkswagen is luring the younger, quirkier customer looking for driving fun. Hyundai offers stylish cars with the longest warranty to attract the conservative consumer looking for value. And if the brand establishes that relationship, fulfills all of its promises, and renews the excitement, it has a customer for life.

The evolving reality is that your patients aren't simply buying dental care - fixed teeth, whiter smiles and things like that. **What they're really buying is you. And a rock solid brand helps you with case acceptance.**

Always remember – you provide a service to your patients that they cannot provide for themselves. You routinely change lives and improve patients' quality of life. That's powerful.

This book will help identify your brand, make it stronger and then give you the tools and mindset you need to dominate your market.

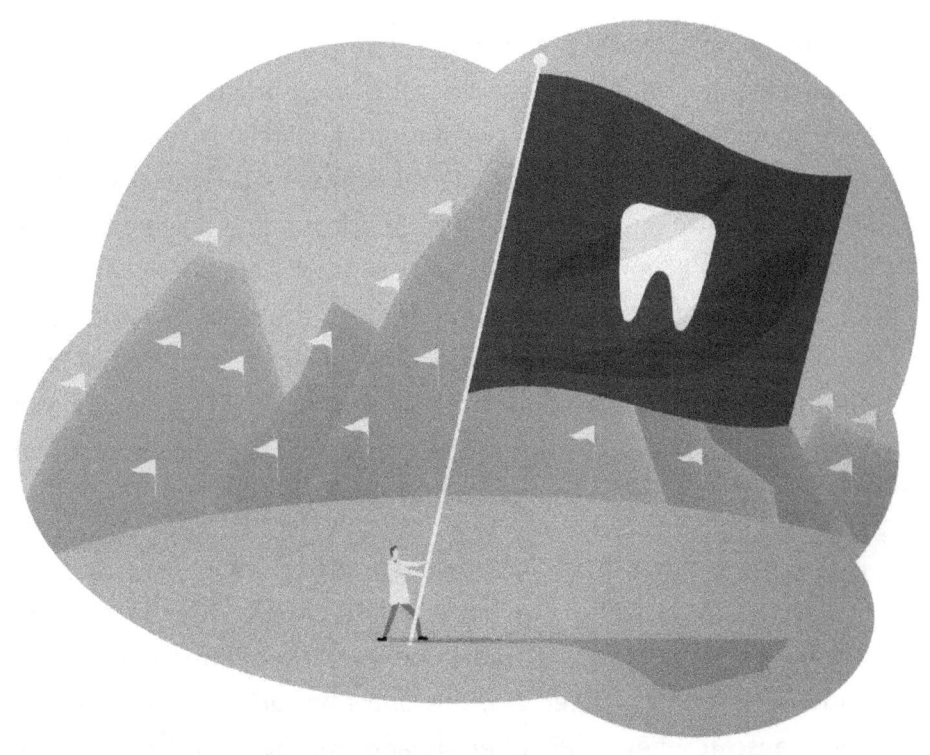

Why Do You Need A Brand?

So far, we've focused a lot on big consumer brands – brands we've all known and loved for several decades. It's easy to see why a beer or a restaurant or a shampoo needs to establish a brand, advertise it, and keep it in the front of consumers' minds. Products are tangible. They're things we use almost every day. They're (generally) consistent in how they are produced. And they're (relatively) easy to promote and advertise. There are so many of them out there that companies have to establish their niche and maintain the relationship with customers. But why would a service-oriented business, such as a dental practice, need a brand?

Mostly for that last reason. And it's a big one.

When you first started practicing, you probably had visions of being a great dentist with your name on the door, practicing in a clean, well-appointed office, with a competent staff and many smiling customers of a certain age or special dental need. And that's how most usually think when they graduate from dental school. It's a start, but it will, in no way, differentiate you from your neighboring dentist down the road, or the hundreds in the area, and compel a patient to walk through your door first. **You need to be noticed.** You need a distinct reason for being. You need to say, loudly and clearly, why you're different and why you're better. Say it over and over. *And you need to deliver on that promise.*

There are so many choices and so many voices shouting at consumers these days. Our TVs, internet, phones, friends...they all create a confusing mix of messages as they relate to consumer options. This one's better. No, this one's better! No, look, try this one 'cause it's new and different and improved and out of this world! Who do we believe? Who do we trust? We trust the brand...the one that connects with us and promises to fulfill our unique needs...the one that fulfills that promise – again and again. Strong brands cut through the clutter.

STATISTIC ALERT

In the 70's, consumers saw 500 advertising messages per day.

In 2014, consumers were exposed to more than 6,000 per day.

You are not only competing with other dentists for attention. You are competing with everything - family vacations, golf clubs, expensive shoes, kids sports teams and more. Pretty much anything that costs $1,000 or more and is not food or shelter is your competition. And most of those things have established, strong brands. **You need to keep up. You need to compete.**

The internet has created arguably the most significant reason why branding is essential...even critical...to the success of medical practices. The internet has empowered a lot of things, but the most significant empowerment went to consumers. Virtually every product is available to purchase at the consumer's fingertips. Every product and service is available to research... and to refute or recommend. And each of us has the power to influence hundreds of friends and neighbors with our rejections or recommendations in one fell swoop with a single Facebook post. If you've developed a robust and effective brand, you'll be able to maximize those 'Likes' and minimize the fallout from any bad reviews.

STATISTIC ALERT

In the good old days of the 80s and 90s, only 10% of people who were dissatisfied with a product or service actually complained about it to someone. Social media has changed the game. Now everyone with an internet connection is a critic... or an ally.

Listen, no one is perfect. Everyone has a bad day or makes a mistake. But there's an art to solving a problem and turning a negative into a positive. Most problems are small and fixable, until they aren't. The easiest and fastest way to solve this is to have an open and honest relationship with your patients where they come to YOU first if they have a problem. If they trust you, they trust your brand and vice versa. Strong brands makes problems fixable...sometimes even fixing them before they become problems.

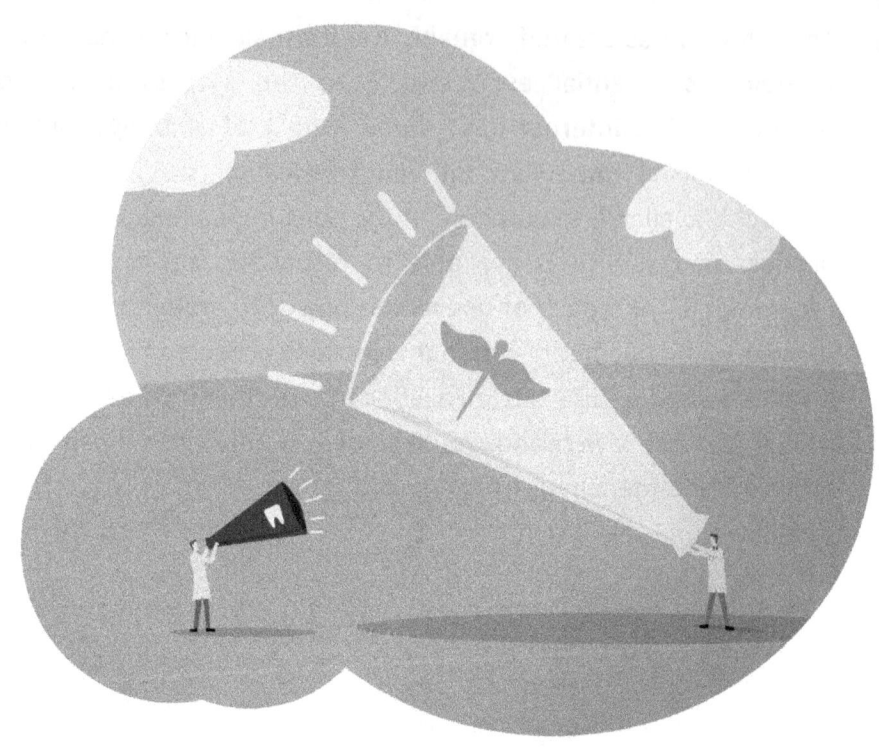

Dentists vs. Physicians

We'd like to point out an important distinction here between physicians and dentists and their relative need for branding. For many reasons, physicians do not tend to brand as heavily as other medical professions. They are often aligned with a larger organization, such as a hospital, that does its own marketing where they enjoy the benefits. Frequently, it's a physician's degree hanging on the wall or his/her published research that 'speaks' for itself and creates brand clout. Most traditional/ general physicians are not sending direct mail pieces, or buying radio ad time or worrying about Facebook followers.

Most patients inherently trust physicians and tend to defer to their expertise and advice. If a physician says to take this medicine or do this therapy or have this procedure done, the vast majority of patients JUST DO IT. They rarely question it, or get a second opinion, or do comparison shopping. They trust what their physician says and they follow the treatment plan.

December 2, 2010

Most Americans Take Doctor's Advice Without Second Opinion

Americans slightly more confident now than in 2002

by Frank Newport

PRINCETON, NJ — Despite the advent of health websites and other widely available sources providing medical research and information, 70% of Americans feel confident in the accuracy of their doctor's advice, and don't feel the need to check for a second opinion or do additional research. Americans' confidence in their doctor is up slightly from eight years ago.

Unfortunately, for whatever reason, dentists don't enjoy the same respect and patient allegiance. Patients go to the dentist and get their semi-annual cleaning and listen to the dentist's treatment recommendations, but they often don't follow them. Perhaps it's because most dental procedures are viewed as cosmetic, not life-saving. Or because going to the dentist is seen as elective instead of compulsory. Maybe it's a lack of understanding of exactly how much education is involved in becoming a good dentist. Or maybe... it's because most dentists have a weak brand or haven't communicated their promise of 'great care' or 'friendly staff' or 'pain-free' or whatever. **Regardless of the reason, wouldn't it be nice if patients just followed a dentist's treatment plan without questioning it?** A strong brand helps to offset this mentality. It enables the dentist to be seen as the trusted care-provider.

In a perfect world, the ADA would become more involved in oral care branding as well. Perhaps if the ADA branded dentistry as well as the National Milk Processor Board branded dairy with the "Got

Milk?" campaign, dentists would see an increase in trust and, ultimately patients.

Ideally, the world will make a paradigm shift in its understanding of how critical dental care is to its overall health. However, until that happens, dentists need to understand how critical branding is to the overall health of their practice.

Branding is essential. Don't underestimate this statement.

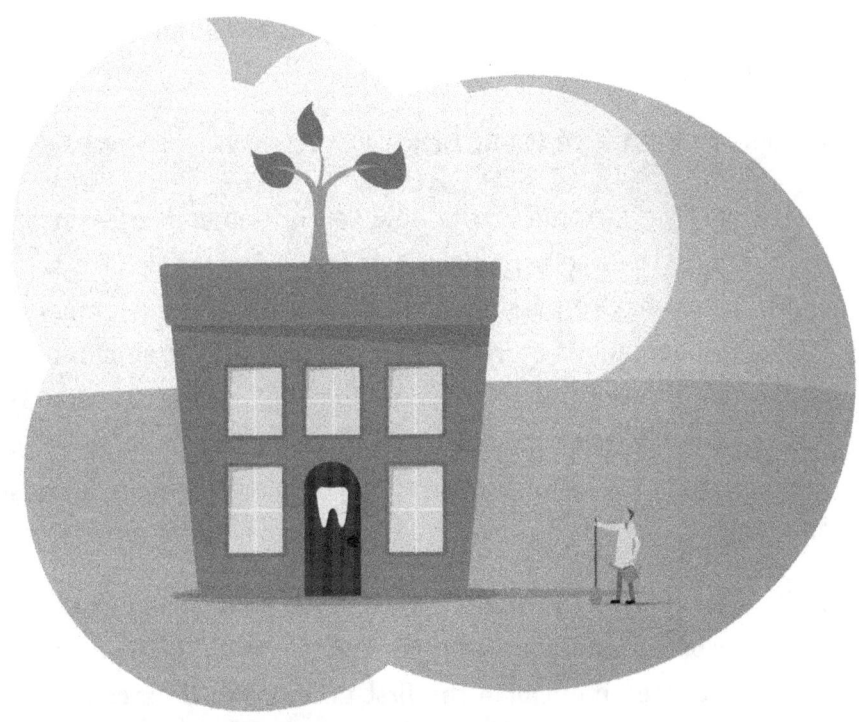

The Benefits Of Branding

A few years ago, a friend stopped into Starbucks for a cup of coffee. Normally, he makes coffee at home and takes it to work in a travel cup, but on this morning, his trusted coffee companion was cracked and leaking. So, he had to stop for coffee on the way to the office. While standing in line at Starbucks, he noticed a display of travel coffee mugs for sale. Without thinking twice or checking the price on the bottom of the cup, he grabbed a silver one and bought it with his coffee. Why would he buy something without checking the price? Why would he buy something without thinking about it first, shopping around, or at least asking a friend? **Because of The Power of The Brand.** To him, Starbucks stands for high quality. They don't sell junk. The brand spoke to him without saying a word and he ended up buying a $20 coffee cup without thinking about it.

Stronger brands not only charge more but make an easier sale. It's that simple.

TIMING + TRUST = TRANSACTION

Last year, Nike introduced the new LeBron James X sneaker at an incredible $315. Nike says their costs for key materials (like cotton) went up, so they're passing along the increase to customers. The fact is, the demand is there, so the price goes up. Premium brands do that kind of thing when no one's looking. *Nike is charging $315 not because it's trying to cover costs, Nike is charging $315 because they can and the market will accept it.* They're running a business – and their strong brand allows them to charge a premium.

What does this mean to you? Make your brand a stronger, more premium brand and your patients will trust you, believe you and accept your treatment plan the first time. **Don't be a commodity. Be different. Be a brand. Be a leader.** Have you considered charging more – not less?

Branding is about developing a relationship – a trusting, evolving, enduring one. Once your patients are there, if you continue to nurture that relationship through your brand, you will have patients for life...and a thriving practice. If you neglect it, your patients will neglect you (or worse...their teeth) and find another dentist who is a better communicator. A better brander.

It's time you had more than just a name on the sign out front. It's time you had a brand – and we're going to show you to do it!

Let's get started.

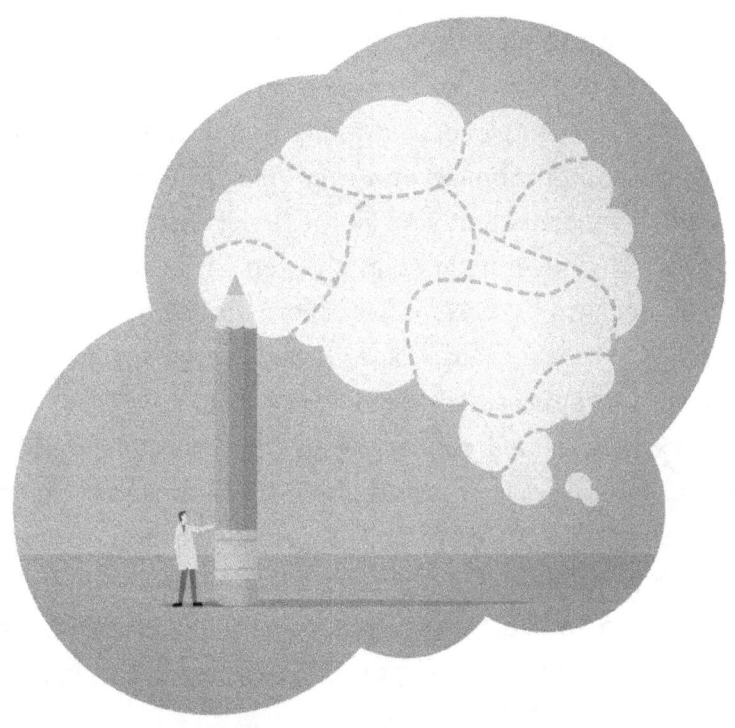

Dissecting A Brand

Ok, so we know what a brand is, what it does, and why we need one, but what is it made of? The simple answer is: **EVERYTHING**. But let us explain.

Many people think of a name and/or a logo when they think of a brand. And while the name and logo are key elements of a brand, they are just a few of the critical parts. Google was considered a terrible, almost laughable, brand name when it was first introduced. And its logo was playful and juvenile...not exactly what you would imagine to be a formidable technology company.

15 years later, Google is one of the largest and fastest growing technology companies, because they stayed true to their initial brand mission: to bring the world together through technology.

They developed a search engine that was user-friendly, inviting, approachable and uniting. They created a corporate campus that is the envy of most employers, offering employees subsidized massages and a sports complex with everything from roller hockey to bocce ball. They consistently make the list of Fortune's Top 100 Employers (landing several times in the top 5). Gmail eclipsed Yahoo! Mail because it was easier, more intuitive, and more comprehensive. Google Maps eclipsed MapQuest because it was more robust, more accessible and more useful. They keep innovating, exciting us and connecting us (the collective world of technology users). Google Glass was one of the most anticipated consumer technologies in years and it does better than bringing information to your fingertips...it creates a shared vision – literally - allowing everyone to see through the same lens. Because they delivered, and continue to deliver, on their brand promise in every initiative, the company has flourished.

Their name, although still rather goofy, became catchy and hip...so much so that it's become a verb in our common internet vernacular. Their logo and look is friendly, approachable, inviting and uniting...just like their search engine...just like their brand. They are consistent in virtually everything they do with their business to achieve the goal of "togetherness through technology". They have connected with us on an entirely different level than any of their competition.

And we trust them. It's the power of branding.

So now let's dissect a brand down to its core elements.

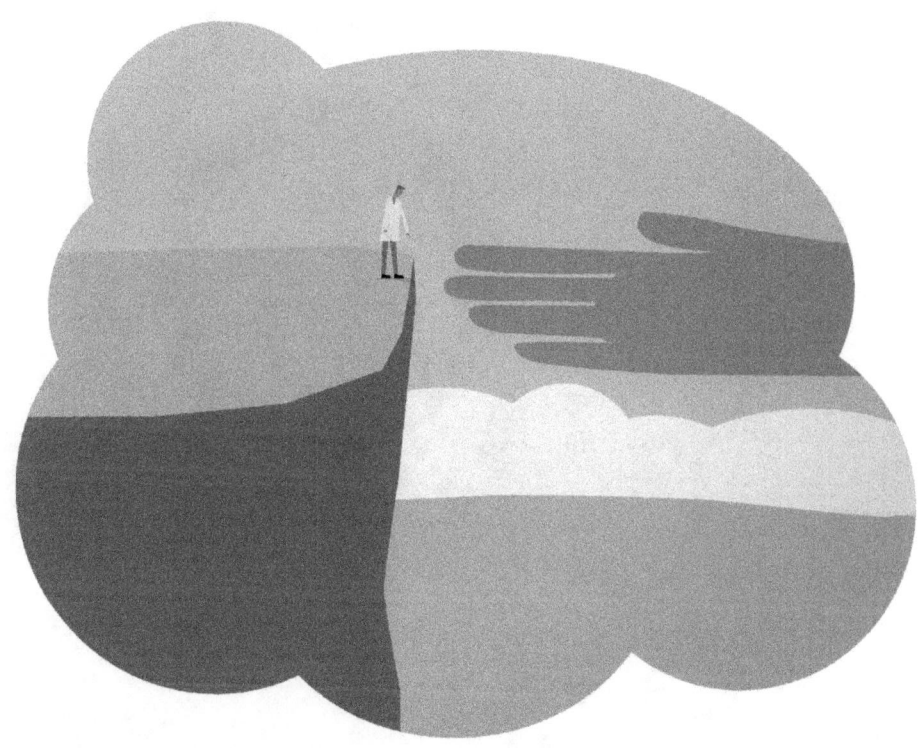

The Fundamental Offer

This is the product or service, at its base level. Google is a search engine. Starbucks is a coffee bar. An iPad is a mobile device. You are a dental practice. There is often nothing unique about it. It's simply the jumping off point. And when you jump, you have to decide who or what you're jumping towards...

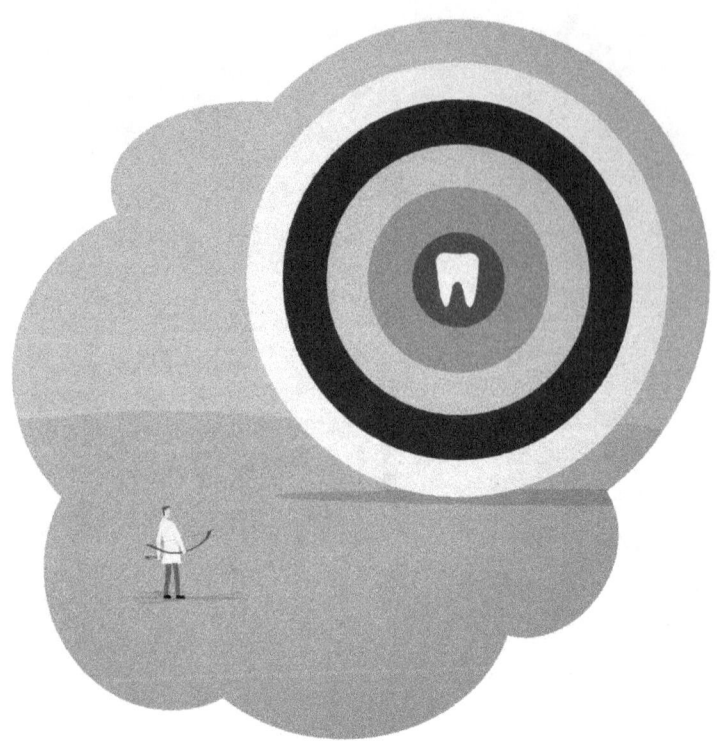

The Target Customer

Imagine a dart board. The entire board represents the possible market of customers for any given product or service. Each smaller ring represents further definition of that market. The goal is to work as far to the center as possible to define that "Bulls-eye Target," also known as your ideal customer.

Starbucks' whole dart board represents all coffee or tea (or smoothie or hot cocoa) drinkers. But they couldn't be consistent in how they delivered their product if they tried to focus on the 12-year-old Swiss-Miss-drinking-Xbox-playing boy, the 30-something-smoothie-slurping-mother-of-4, and the 65-year-old-tea-sipping-grandfather. Their approach to the business would be all over the place. So, instead, they began by focusing on 25-40-year-old urban professionals as their bulls-eye market, basing every business decision on how they believed those particular people would respond. And it worked. When you picture a Starbucks in your mind, who do you see as the patrons? They're most likely men and women in their 30s, on the way to work or working on a laptop. Sure, now that the brand is established (some say ubiquitous), the boy, the mom and the granddad might still stop in for the random offering of smoothies or hot cocoa. But those customers are the icing on the branding cake for Starbucks.

As a dentist, you need to define your target...your ideal patient. It's too hard to be all things to all people. There are pediatric dentists targeting kids and their parents. There are cosmetic dentists targeting yoga moms. But even a general practitioner has his or her specific ideal customer.

Your audience is the group of people most likely to buy your service and the group that you are most capable of serving. So who do you want to target? And please don't say everyone with teeth.

First, start thinking beyond geography. Your target audience is not just those within a 10 mile radius of your practice. We know several dentists who have patients that have moved out of state, but still drive hours or get on a plane to see them. **Their service and brand are that strong.**

Your target may begin with a dental specialization. It may be based on demographics – age, income, healthcare profile, geography, etc. Whatever it is, your brand should focus on that ideal bulls-eye target. Is it male or female? What age is she? How does he behave? How does she pay? Is he a techie? Is she extremely health-conscious? If you can define and attract that customer and fulfill your brand promise, your practice will expand from there. Targeting a specific audience allows you to speak consistently, so you don't dilute your message trying to appeal to the masses. You'll get those "icing" patients as well, but to be true to your brand, you have to know exactly who you're talking to.

And now to find just the right talking points...

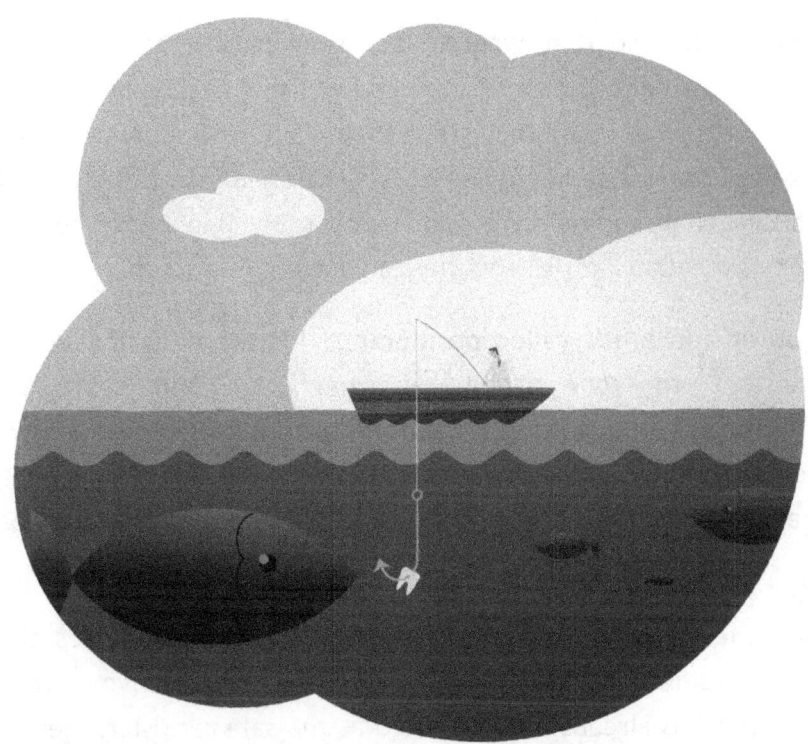

The Positioning

What's your hook?

So you've figured out exactly WHO you want as your patients. Now you need to figure out WHAT is most important to them, and "position" yourself to be able to fulfill their needs.

Let's revisit the car industry. If you asked every car company if their cars are safe, reliable, cutting-edge, high-performing, etc., each would say yes to everything without blinking an eye. And they may be right – the cars themselves might be all of those things. But *brands* can't be all things to all people. It's too confusing. It doesn't allow a consumer to identify with one product or service over another. So car brands carve their niche.

They decide who they want to buy their cars. They determine what's most important to those people. They decide which needs aren't being met. And they stake their claim with a brand. BMW picked performance and owns it. Volvo picked safety and owns it. Volkswagen picked quirky fun and owns it. Hyundai picked sensible practicality. Cadillac picked American luxury. And so on...

In brand-speak, it's called positioning. It's the thing that's most important to your target customers. It's the thing that differentiates you from your competitors. It's what you promise and consistently fulfill. It's what they remember you for. And it's what they trust they'll get every time they set foot in your practice.

Often times, the first person to claim something is the one remembered by the consumer. If you think about Mercedes, they make incredibly safe cars (maybe even safer than a Volvo), but the consumer has already labeled Volvo as *the* safe car. Mercedes can try and claim it, but Volvo (if they continue to brand as well as they have) will always be first in the consumer's mind.

Most dentists will, by default or by accident, position themselves as the one providing great care. But if everybody is claiming it, and most are achieving it, why would a patient have any reason to choose one dentist over another? They might as well throw a dart at a map. Great care should be a given in a medical profession. You need to figure out what it is about your practice's individual experience that makes it truly *different*...and better.

Here are some examples of brand positioning options that a dental practice might claim:

- On the Cutting Edge / State-of-the-Art Technology
- Family Focused
- Providing an Enjoyable/Fun Experience
- Incredible Customer Relations/Service
- Most Experienced/Knowledgeable Clinicians
- Community Oriented
- TMJ/Headache Specialist
- Physical Comfort - Pain-free Dentistry / Sedation / Sleep Solutions

Like the car companies, you may be several, or even all, of these things. But to be remembered and revered you have to claim one as your own. **Target your customer. Find a position. Own it. And get ready to prove that you own it...**

Exercise #1 – Positioning Statement

Now try drafting your own unique positioning statement. Using a template to clearly define your positioning statement can be helpful:

For ____(Target Customer)____, that __(Needs / Reason to Buy)__,

the ____(Business Name)____ is a ___(Category / Description)____

that provides _(Key Benefit / Promise)_____.

Unlike _____(Main Competitors)___, _____(Business Name)_____

is _____(Unique Differentiator)_____.

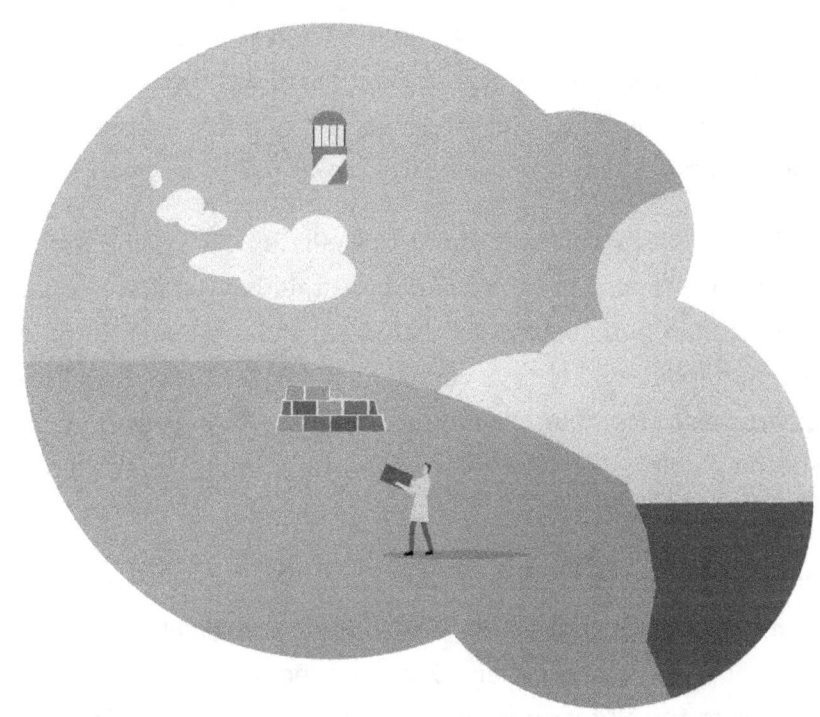

Features & Benefits

Just because you claim to be the most tech-savvy or customer-friendly practice in your greater metro area, does not mean that people will simply take your word for it. You have to back it up with the goods – the tangible evidence that you are who you say you are, that you do what you say you do. You have to provide features and benefits as that first round of proof.

Features are the tangible things that make your product or service great, and the benefits are why those things are important and desirable to your target customers – why they will seek you out and come back for more. Google's *features* were speed, ease, reach, intuitiveness. Their customers *benefitted* with efficiency, accessibility, knowledge and connectedness. Starbucks' *features* were made-to-order coffee, inviting environments and superb service. Customers enjoyed the *benefits* of a consistently great cup of coffee coupled with feelings of comfort, familiarity and specialness.

Let's imagine a cosmetic dentist...we'll call him Phil Young. He wants his practice to be a relaxing destination – a place adults are comfortable and relaxed to visit...even more frequently than the recommended two times a year. So he decides to create a luxurious environment complete with *features* like free premium coffee, soothing colors, iPads in every operatory, and a service-oriented, enthusiastic staff.

Product brands usually have an easier time than service brands touting features because of their inherent tangibility. They can be held, applied, eaten, driven, worn, poured, played, sat on, etc. etc. It's easier to sell features and benefits for product brands because they are generally more obvious, easily controlled and quantifiable. When Philips designs, develops and manufactures a Sonicare toothbrush, each step is in the company's control, each feature is carefully defined, and what we purchase is a fixed item.

Service features are typically more unwieldy, with a greater number of moving parts and influences beyond the brand owner's control (and by 'moving parts', we usually mean the people actually carrying out the service). When fast food Mexican restaurant Chipotle opens a new retail store, they are formulaic about environmental design, supplies, recipe formula and rigorous and consistent employee training. But they can never fully control how each server prepares a burrito or how each cashier interacts with a customer. **Staff will always be a variable.**

Your dental practice, since it falls in the "service" realm, needs to be very deliberate in how it defines and manages its features. Remember Phil? If he positions his practice as a professional destination and has all the right equipment and service, but the receptionist is snarky and the hygienist is glum, the brand falls apart. Your people are your greatest asset, but also your greatest liability. They personify the service, bringing the brand to life. It's a good idea to decide exactly what type of *personality* you want your brand to have before you hire and train new, or re-train existing, employees. **Everyone and everything in your practice affects your brand – and, in turn, affects the patient experience.** Start with your online presence, phone etiquette, outdoor signage, lobby environment, paint on the walls, receptionist, operatory equipment, dress code, lighting, music and more. Literally everything affects your brand either positively or negatively.

Make sure that everyone in your practice believes in you and your brand. If they don't, your brand won't have a fighting chance.

Exercise #2 – Features & Benefits

Take some time to think about what features of a dental practice
are important to your customers. Then consider which are most
important to you, your particular practice and to differentiating you
from your competition. Make a list and then think about what the
actual benefit is to patients. REMEMBER THE BENEFITS. Make
them part of your daily vernacular. Speak in benefits...they're what
persuade. They're what sell. They're what create loyalty.

	Features	Benefits
1		
2		
3		
4		
5		
6		

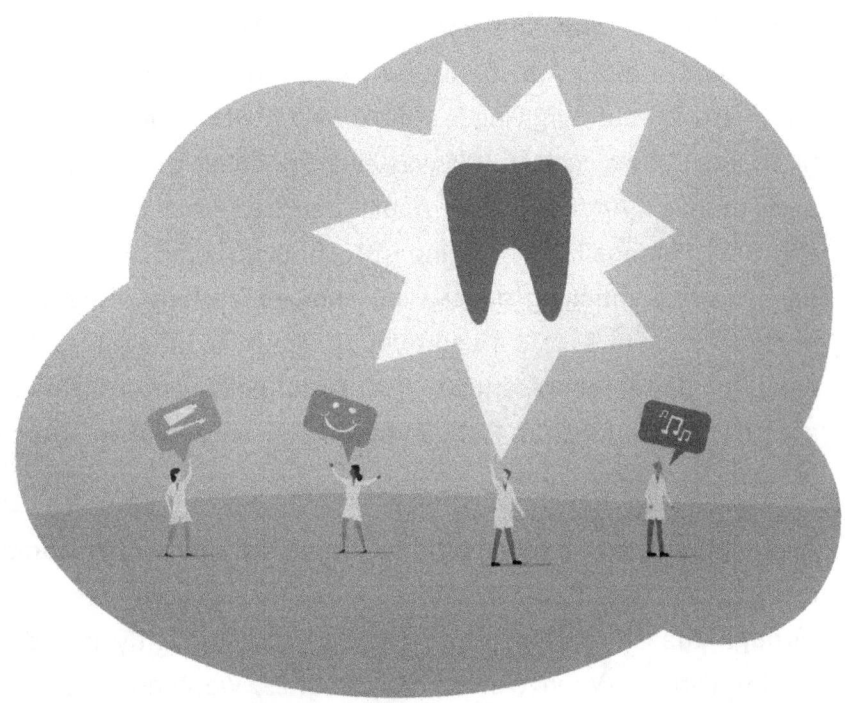

The Personality

Branding itself is a difficult concept for many people to grasp. It might seem like fluff or smoke and mirrors at first, but we've shown why it is so critical to boosting a business's bottom line. But now you might think we're getting even fluffier by talking about brand personality. However, personality is what ties it all together...what creates that consistent brand voice...and what will ultimately make your customers listen and keep listening.

To illustrate, let's jump into the decades-long war in the computer industry: Mac vs. PC. In 1984, the Macintosh computer was introduced as the user-friendly alternative to the PC. It was successfully marketed to be used in homes, schools and for creative/design work. While PCs continued to innovate, a decade later the Macintosh lagged and market share declined. And that's when the real branding began. In 1998, Apple rebooted and redesigned the Macintosh, not only by overhauling the technology and features, but by giving it a personality with iMac. It had a fun nickname! It was colorful! It was even friendlier to use! It was hip and creative! And with that, Apple launched what would become the most personality-driven line of technology ever. Even some of their most compelling advertising showed nothing more than a person ("Hi, I'm Mac"...a cool, young, smart, confident, laid-back creative dude) representing the technology and outsmarting another person ("Hi, I'm PC"...an older, dull, conservative, insecure, business geek) every time.

Apple infuses personality into its brand at every opportunity – through its late founder, Steve Jobs, through the technology, through the advertising, even through their recently introduced Apple Watch. When we use our iPhones, we channel our cool, young, smart, creative selves and it makes us feel more confident. And that's the powerful effect of brand personality.

When most people think of their visits to the dentist's office, they usually jump straight to the chair. They remember the conversation they had with the hygienist and then recall the scraping, drilling and suction noises imposed by the dentist. And that's because most dental practices haven't branded themselves at all; they haven't taken the initiative to infuse personality beyond that of the dentist.

If you don't create a brand, then you're just another mouth mechanic whom patients will dread seeing. Speaking of mechanics, think about how you feel when you take your car in for service. Many people feel a sense of uncertainty and anxiety. Is my car ok? How long will this take? How much is this going to cost me? But those that trust the brand of their car and "their guy" in the service department don't experience that same dread. Those that go to a service department where there is a friendly staff, fresh coffee, television, clean environment, up-to-date magazines and a shuttle to shopping might actually enjoy the visit. Brands replace uncertainty with confidence, anxiety with anticipation.

Your brand personality should shine through the colors on the walls, the music, the posts on your Facebook page and the greetings of the receptionist. Your marketing (be it newspaper advertisements, appointment reminder cards, your website or radio ads, etc.) should all sing from the same hymn sheet, using the same voice and reiterating the same messages.(More on that later)

It's time to mention something very critical: **The dentist is the most important asset of a dental brand.** Even if you are part of a larger organization or in a co-branded group of dental practices, you (as the dentist), will have the greatest influence on how your existing (and potential) patients perceive your brand.

And with great influence comes great responsibility. You must decide on a brand personality that is not counter to your own disposition. If you are reserved, mild-mannered and conservative in the way you provide treatment, nobody is going to buy that your practice is bold, modern and cutting edge just because you blare hip-hop from your sound system and cover your walls in various animal prints. Consumers are savvy. And they can spot a phony even before you recline their chair. Your dental brand will never be credible if the dentist doesn't have the personality to back it up. We're not saying that you shouldn't push yourself to embody a great brand concept. We're just saying to be realistic about what you, and your natural personality, can achieve. Be yourself...and highlight the best version of yourself.

So the brand personality should reflect the dentist's. But what about all of the other personalities in the office? How can a practice's brand embody one personality when there are so many 'persons' involved in running the office? We're not saying that your receptionist, office manager and hygienist need to check their own personalities at the door and act differently all day. But how they answer the phone, how they greet and treat patients, how they dress, etc., will have a significant impact on how a patient experiences your brand. It should all be consistent and it should become second-nature…and, thus, genuine.

We're sure that you have effective hiring and customer service training in place already. But if you can orient your customer service so that it brings your brand personality to life, it will help to make the rest of the branding process seamless.

Your patients want to feel comfortable and **they want to like you.**

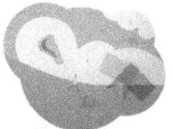

Listen

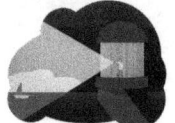

See

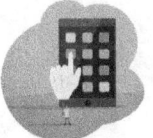

Touch

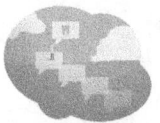

Speak

4 'SENSIBLE' STEPS TO CREATING A COMPELLING BRAND

Now that we understand the importance of a brand and the components that make one up, where do we go from here? A helpful way to approach branding is to think about it as a 'sensory' process. Because your brand should be a part of everything you do, you should use all of your senses when building it, and your customer should use all of his or her senses when experiencing it. We're going to focus on 4 sensory steps for you to implement as you create your brand: Listening, Seeing, Touching, and Speaking.

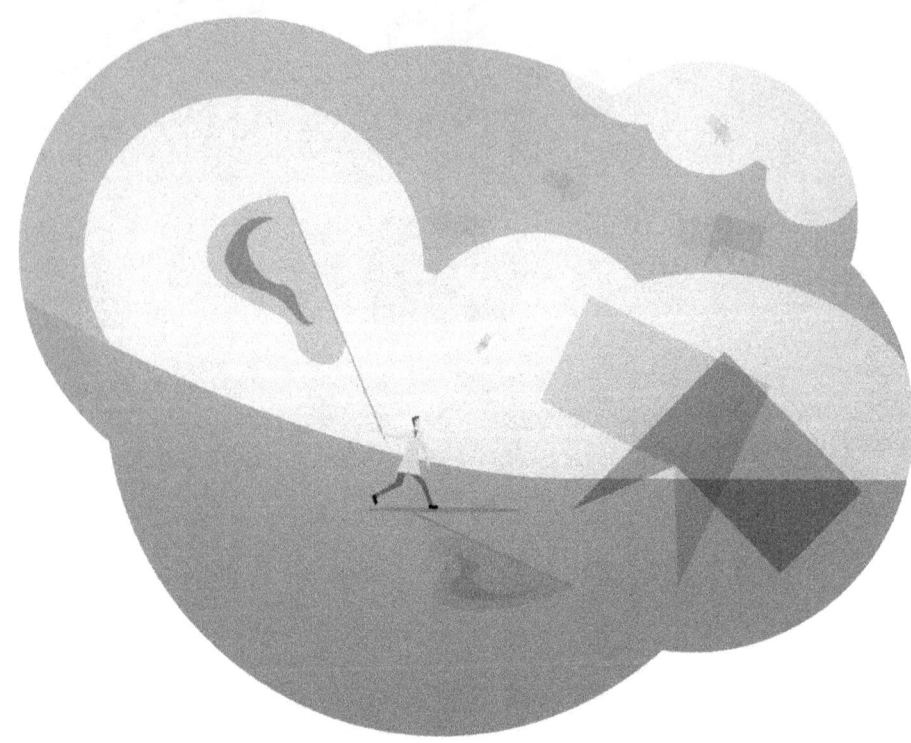

Listen

(...to your customers, to your staff, to your market)

So you probably subscribe to all the right dental publications, read peer reviewed articles and go to a study club and think you have your finger on the pulse of the industry. You might send out "How Did We Do?" surveys to patients the day after their appointment and believe you truly know how you're doing. Maybe you even stake out the competition to see what they're doing that you should be doing too. And all of those things are valuable. But you need both a finger on the pulse and an ear to the ground. While a finger on the pulse tells you what's happening now, an ear to the ground tells you what's going to happen in the future...the ear brings the real value that will enable your practice to capitalize on upcoming trends and flourish. So listen up.

Listening to Your Customers

There are competent marketers and there are brilliant marketers. Competent marketers might be wildly creative advertising guys or scholarly executives that know every sales figure in every region down to the decimal. But most marketers don't ever take the time to truly listen to what's going on...to hear their audience and discern why that hilarious ad isn't selling products, or why those sales numbers aren't shifting in the right direction. Brilliant marketers do.

Brilliant marketers care more about listening to their target audience than they do about talking to them. Brilliant marketers don't just skim through and file away complaints; they delve deeper, reading between the lines to discern what their audience is really saying. And they take that feedback or "customer insight" and apply it to everything they're doing with their brand. Defined, 'customer insight' is "the collection, deployment and *interpretation* of information that allows a business to acquire, *develop* and retain their customers." Interpretation. Development. Those are the operative words. And we'll explain why

We've talked about your target audience and how you should define it. Now, we're talking about how, once you define it, your audience should define you...and how you market your practice.

Let's say that you've decided your bulls-eye target is a 40-year-old married mother of 2, who works part-time, has a household income of $100k, has health and dental insurance, does yoga 4 times a week, and is active on social media. Whether you are just starting your practice, or you are a 30-year veteran, you need to talk to her (to 10 of her if you can get to them), and find out what she is looking for in her dentist experience. What's the environment like? What's the personality of the staff? What is the style of the dentist? How is she cared for? How should the office communicate with her, before, during, and after the appointment?

Everyone knows that women make almost all of the healthcare decisions in the household. Target them. Listen to them. Cater to them.

Some practitioners might develop a quick one-page survey to send out via email or through social media. Some might set up an iPad in the waiting area with a 3-minute survey. Some might take a more casual approach and have regular face-to-face conversations with existing patients and friends and neighbors that fall in that target audience. And this isn't just a "patient experience survey" where they tell you how much they liked or disliked their last visit to the dentist. This is a survey where they get to think about and relay their *ideal* experience, no holds barred. There are many ways to talk with your audience. Find one that works with your style and your routine. You'd be surprised how many people will want to help you – and you'll probably be surprised by their answers.

Document your conversations. Listen again. Pull out great ideas. Expand on them. Listen again...and more. Say thank you. Any insight you can gain by listening to your ideal customers is invaluable to developing a strong and enduring brand. And always keep that conversation flowing.

Listening To Employees

There's another blunder that the 'competent marketer' often makes: only paying attention to the immediate customer when making business or marketing decisions. We've just told you that customer insight is invaluable – and it is; but it's not the only song you should be dancing to. The 'brilliant marketer' also hears beyond his or her customers. There are so many opportunities to learn how to improve your business and develop a compelling brand. And once you start to see them (and hear them), they seem so obvious.

First let's point out your greatest informational resource – your staff. Many business owners and marketers overlook the insight and knowledge that employees can impart. They're the ones on the front line. They're the ones in constant contact with customers, hearing feedback, solving problems. They're often the ones with the panoramic view of the office, the environment, the market. They compile a wealth of invaluable information and they often have the insight to know how to create solutions and opportunities in the business. Tap into it. Not only will you gain a whole heap of knowledge, you will also empower your employees by letting them know they have a voice in running the business and are essential to the success of the practice. They're more invested and happier. You're smarter and more effective. You're both more productive and fulfilled.

Disney is an example of a company that empowers its employees by giving them an active role in shaping the business and the brand. Every mouse, duck and princess that greets patrons at their theme parks is trained to collect customer feedback and provide insight to management that is used to improve processes, products and, ultimately, profits. They hire cast members based on their penchant for creativity and innovation...not only in their acting role, but in how they can contribute to enhancing the brand. Employees truly feel they are an integral part of the family. And that, in our estimation, is a big part of what brings the true magic to Disney's brand promise of "magical family fun".

Listening to the Market

The final sounds you should be hearing are those of the market that you're in. It may seem obvious, but you should always be aware of what's going on around you. Particularly in service businesses, we get very comfortable in our own environments and routines. We spend 8-10 hours a day in the same restaurant, store or office. We rarely venture out. We do our jobs and try to do them well. We have a reasonably steady flow of loyal customers. *And if mediocre is your goal, then stay the course!*

However, if challenge, stimulation, growth and increasing success are your goals, you have to get out and experience the great big world. You have to know and understand the trends in your industry. You have to know your competition intimately. Without that knowledge, you miss every opportunity to develop your business and your brand.

So, in the great big dental world, you should read those industry magazines, meet with your colleagues to discuss best practices, read blogs (and write your own), and continue that continuing education. Pay attention to technology trends, be familiar with the latest gadgets (even if you don't buy them), and be able to speak about emerging treatment techniques (even if they're not in your specialization). The more you know about the evolving world of dentistry, the more you'll be inspired to grow, and the more you'll inspire your brand.

Keep your friends close and your competition closer. Know what makes Dr. Millenial's practices better than yours. And know where they aren't measuring up. You, or one of your staff, might even try becoming the patient. Experience your own office from the patient's point of view. Visit other offices and experience the service, the environment, the equipment, the care, the follow up. Compare the experiences and find the gaps. Every time you can identify what your competition isn't doing well, you create an opportunity to do even better. It allows you to differentiate your brand by filling the unfulfilled needs of potential patients.

So we hope you've *heard* what we're saying: Listen to your customers. Listen to your staff. Listen to the market. Listen to colleagues you meet at seminars and tradeshows. And if you truly hear them, you'll gain the knowledge and insight you need to innovate your practice and inspire your brand.

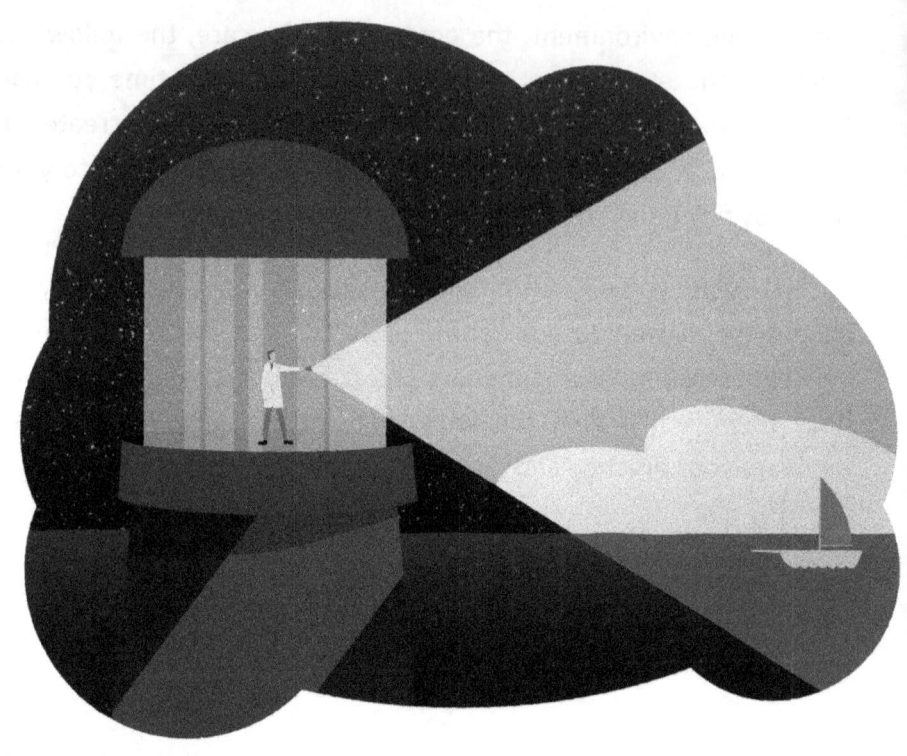

See

(...where you want to be)

Now that you've listened intently, and you know what opportunities lie ahead, you need to seize them (or SEE-z them). You need to create your vision for your practice.

We've talked about brand positioning. That's the first step in creating the vision. It's the overarching goal of where you want to be. It's the promise you deliver to your patients...again and again. Do you want to be the most innovative practice? Do you want to be the friendliest? Do you want to be the 'family' dentist? Do you want to be the very best clinician who speaks and lectures around the world?

How do you decide what position to take?

First, go back to what you heard. What did your target customers tell you they needed most? Maybe they want cutting edge technology and treatment. Maybe comfort, familiarity and trust of the dentist are most important. Maybe it's efficiency and practicality they need. Find the need and then look at what your competitors are doing (and not doing). You're bound to find a gap...and there is your opportunity. There is the first glimpse of your overall vision.

Your brand positioning not only differentiates you from your competitors, it gives you a defined purpose. And if you fulfill that purpose, you become an authority. Authorities are trusted. Trust builds relationships. And relationships mean customers for life.

Let's talk about one of the great modern visionaries in terms of branding and marketing: Richard Branson. He decided as a teenager that entrepreneurialism was his calling. As do most entrepreneurs, he failed early and often and even landed in jail, but his vision kept him going...through the music, airline, telecommunications, hospitality and financial industries.

Branson is always looking ahead, seeing where he next wants to be. He takes risks and sometimes those risks don't pay off, but more often they do. He is about creativity, follow-through and making a difference in people's lives. And his own vision and values are clearly articulated in the company's:

> "Virgin believes in making a difference. We stand for value
> for money, quality, innovation, fun and a sense of
> competitive challenge. We strive to achieve this by
> empowering our employees to continually deliver an
> unbeatable customer experience...

Virgin Group companies are part of one big family rather than a hierarchy. They are empowered to run their own affairs, yet the companies actively help one another...

At our core we believe business must be a force for good and use its influence and resources to help find solutions to some of the world's major issues. "

Vision keeps you inspired and focused. It might not get you to $4.6 billion in net-worth, but it's what you need for your business, and your brand, to succeed and grow.

Find your vision and keep it in the front of your mind in everything you do.

Starbuck's Mission, Vision & Values

Mission Statement: To inspire and nurture the human spirit – one person, one cup and one neighborhood at a time.

Our Coffee

It has always been, and will always be, about quality. We're passionate about ethically sourcing the finest coffee beans, roasting them with great care, and improving the lives of people who grow them. We care deeply about all of this; our work is never done.

Our Partners

We're called partners, because it's not just a job, it's our passion. Together, we embrace diversity to create a place where each of us can be ourselves. We always treat each other with respect and dignity. And we hold each other to that standard.

Our Customers

When we are fully engaged, we connect with, laugh with, and uplift the lives of our customers – even if just for a few moments. Sure, it starts with the promise of a perfectly made beverage, but our work goes far beyond that. It's really about human connection.

Our Stores

When our customers feel this sense of belonging, our stores become a haven, a break from the worries outside, a place where you can meet with friends. It's about enjoyment at the speed of life – sometimes slow and savored, sometimes faster. Always full of humanity.

Our Neighborhood

Every store is part of a community, and we take our responsibility to be good neighbors seriously. We want to be invited in wherever we do business. We can be a force for positive action bringing together our partners, customers, and the community to contribute every day. Now we see that our responsibility and our potential for good is even larger. The world is looking to Starbucks to set the new standard, yet again. We will lead.

Our Shareholders

We know that as we deliver in each of these areas, we enjoy the kind of success that rewards our shareholders. We are fully accountable to get each of these elements right so that Starbucks – and everyone it touches – can endure and thrive.

Mayo Clinic Mission and Values

Mission: To inspire hope and contribute to health and well-being by providing the best care to every patient through integrated clinical practice, education and research.

Primary Value: The needs of the patient come first.

Value statements:

Respect
Treat everyone in our diverse community, including patients, their families and colleagues, with dignity.

Compassion
Provide the best care, treating patients and family members with sensitivity and empathy.

Integrity
Adhere to the highest standards of professionalism, ethics and personal responsibility, worthy of the trust our patients place in us.

Healing
Inspire hope and nurture the well-being of the whole person, respecting physical, emotional and spiritual needs.

Teamwork
Value the contributions of all, blending the skills of individual staff members in unsurpassed collaboration.

Excellence
Deliver the best outcomes and highest quality service through the dedicated effort of every team member.

Innovation
Infuse and energize the organization, enhancing the lives of those we serve, through the creative ideas and unique talents of each employee.

Stewardship
Sustain and reinvest in our mission and extended communities by wisely managing our human, natural and material resources.

EXERCISE #3 – YOUR MISSION

Now it's time to get interactive. Let's write out your mission statement and vision statement as well as your core values.

Your mission statement is rock solid – it is the over-arching reason you do what you do – it NEVER changes.

Your vision statement is aspirational and dynamic– it can evolve as you change, your practice changes and your patients change. For example, if you invest in digital dentistry, this could change your vision to provide a standard of care that is both better and more convenient.

Your Mission, Vision and Values define you.

What do you believe in?

Our Practice's Mission (our reason for being) is to _____

_____

_____

_____

_____

Our Vision (what we aspire to be in the eyes of our patients) is to _

_____

_____

_____

_____

Our Values (what inspire us and guide our behavior) are _____

_____

_____

_____

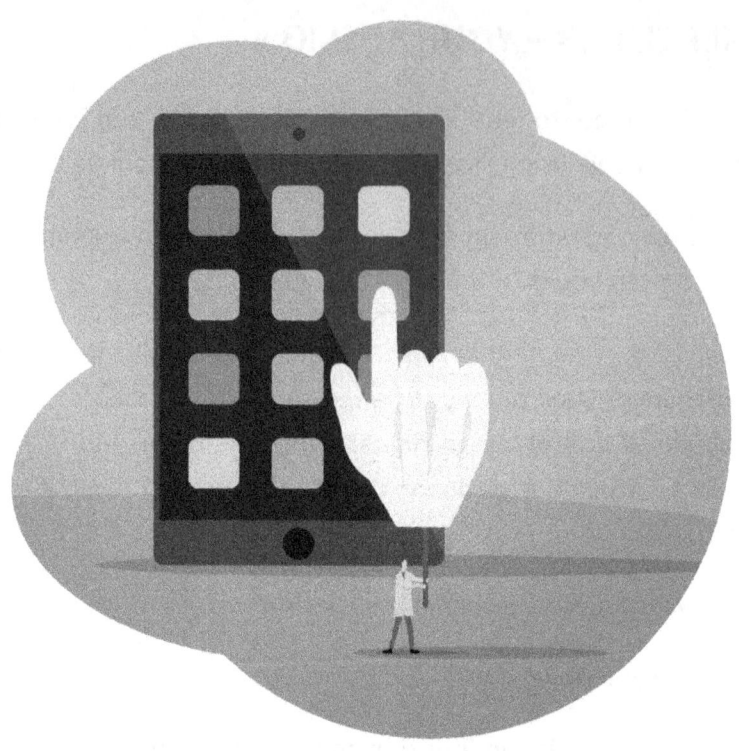

Touch

(Connect through every point of contact)

You see the big picture. You've picked who and what you want to be. Now you need to own it. And prove that you own it in every 'touch-point' of your practice – i.e. connect your audience to your brand through everything that touches them -emotionally, physically or mentally. Connect through the lobby environment, the paint colors, the website, the YouTube channel, the chair, the equipment, the demeanor of the receptionist, the banter with the hygienist, the follow-up emails. A vision is just a mirage until you put tangible evidence in place. Then vision becomes reality.

Let's look at Nordstrom for a moment. When John Nordstrom founded the company a century ago, he had a vision of owning the 'customer service' positioning. And he made it a reality. Not just because Nordstrom has friendly, attentive sales representatives. Its customer service permeates every aspect of the company - the store environment, the employees, the merchandise, the restaurants, the marketing, etc. It is evident in every touch-point, in every interaction.

The store environment is all about fulfilling the customer experience. Live piano music; perfectly orchestrated scents and airflow; soothing lighting; inviting restaurants. It's all meant to create a pleasurable shopping experience, yet not so relaxing that customers forget to shop.

Even their sales are designed to make the customer feel special and a sense of belonging. They have two annual sales that rarely fall in the traditional retail sale cycle, thus making customers feel they are members of a special club.

Their salespeople are trained and empowered to do whatever is necessary to ensure that the customer is not only always right, but always fulfilled. They honor returns on anything, anytime. They deliver merchandise to customers' houses. They open the store after hours for customer 'emergencies'. They introduce themselves and often hand out business cards so they become names, not just faces. They are trained to read the customer to know how to tailor their approach to the individual on the sales floor. Employees are empowered, in their initial orientation, to make decisions based on their best judgment (exhibit A: 1-sheet employee "handbook" on next page).

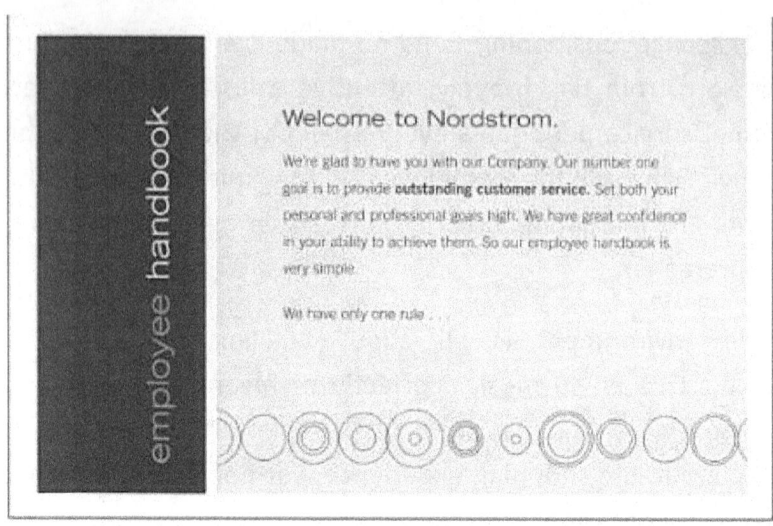

Welcome to Nordstrom.

We're glad to have you with our Company. Our number one goal is to provide **outstanding customer service.** Set both your personal and professional goals high. We have great confidence in your ability to achieve them. So our employee handbook is very simple.

We have only one rule . .

(Turning over the card)

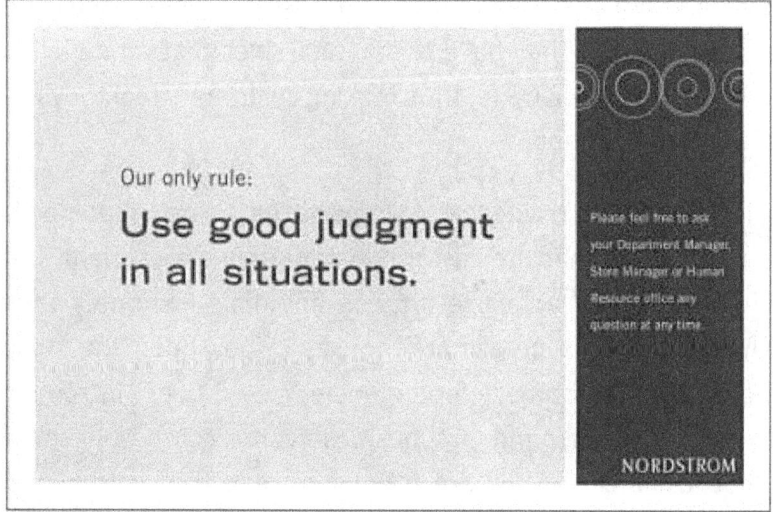

Our only rule:

Use good judgment in all situations.

Please feel free to ask your Department Manager, Store Manager or Human Resource office any question at any time.

NORDSTROM

Everything Nordstrom does is in an effort to make the customer feel special so that they will return again and again. And each time they will pay more for their clothes, their shoes, their perfumes because the experience is worth it. It's not for everyone, but it's exactly, perfectly right for their target demographic.

The brand that touches is the brand that connects.

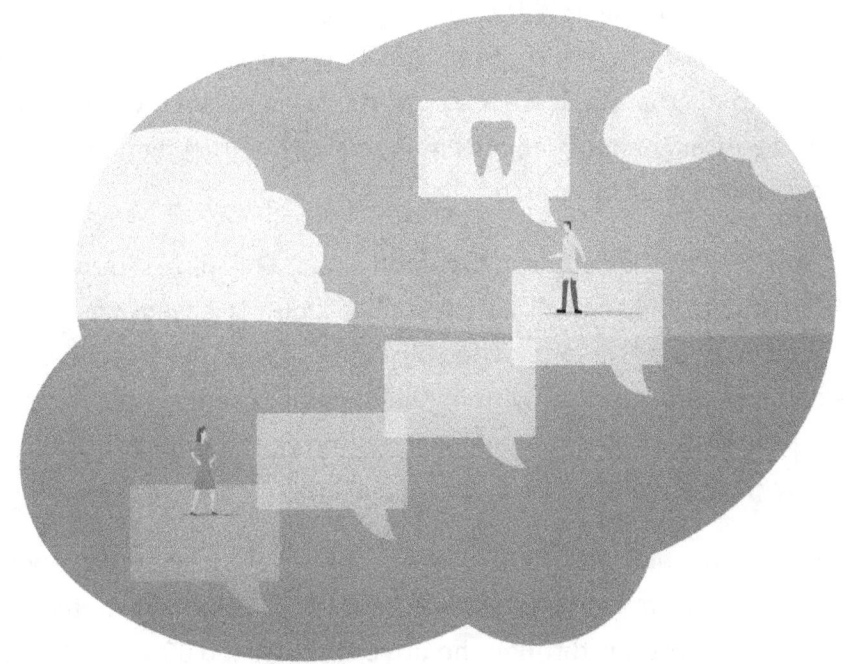

Speak

(...your brand in everything you say)

In business, whether we're talking, writing, emailing, advertising, telemarketing, blogging, promoting, attending tradeshows, or direct mailing, we are always attempting to speak to our potential customers. That's why it's called 'Marketing Communications'. We are constantly trying to communicate the benefit of our offering. Speech, while not one of the traditional 5 senses, is the faculty we use in marketing to incite all of the other senses, and ultimately motivate a purchase.

So it's critical that when we speak to our target audience, we make sure our brand and its position and personality are consistent in everything we say. How we speak is, in large part, what dictates the nature of our relationships - personally and professionally. If we're moody or unpredictable in how we communicate, people tend to distrust us. If we are consistent and reliable, we earn trust. And trust is the most important element to attracting and retaining customers in all businesses.

Let's look at the southern fast-food chain, Chik-fil-A. Founded by a Christian family, much of their philosophy is based on Christian principles and "servant leadership". The idea is that if leaders serve and speak to the staff with humility, compassion, genuineness and a passion for service, employees will serve customers in the same way. And it works.

Visit a Chik-fil-A and you'll probably be greeted at the door with a friendly welcome. After you receive your order promptly (their goal is 90 seconds through the drive-through and 60 seconds at the counter) and you say, "Thank you," your server will say, "My pleasure". And after you've sat down, a manager might visit your table to ask how things are. And when you say, "Just fine, thank you", they'll respond, "My pleasure." "My pleasure" is thought to be more classy and distinctive, associated with higher levels of service than a plain old "You're welcome". It's what each Chik-fil-A employee is trained to say and it elevates the service in customer's minds. Chik-fil-A customers are confident that they will be treated with compassion, humility and genuineness. And they've been doing it this way for over 50 years – way ahead of the curve.

It's just one example of how a business that speaks consistently to its customers creates a better customer experience and brings its brand to life. We're not saying that you need to create a script for your employees or post "Lingo Laws" on the wall, but you do need to decide what voice and demeanor you will use every time you speak to your customers.

Speak to your existing patients. Speak to your target audience. Speak through advertising, social media, promotions, public relations, online marketing and through your own mouth. **Patients are NOT buying dental care. Patients are buying YOU! They're buying your brand.** Speak your brand loud and clear. And patients will listen.

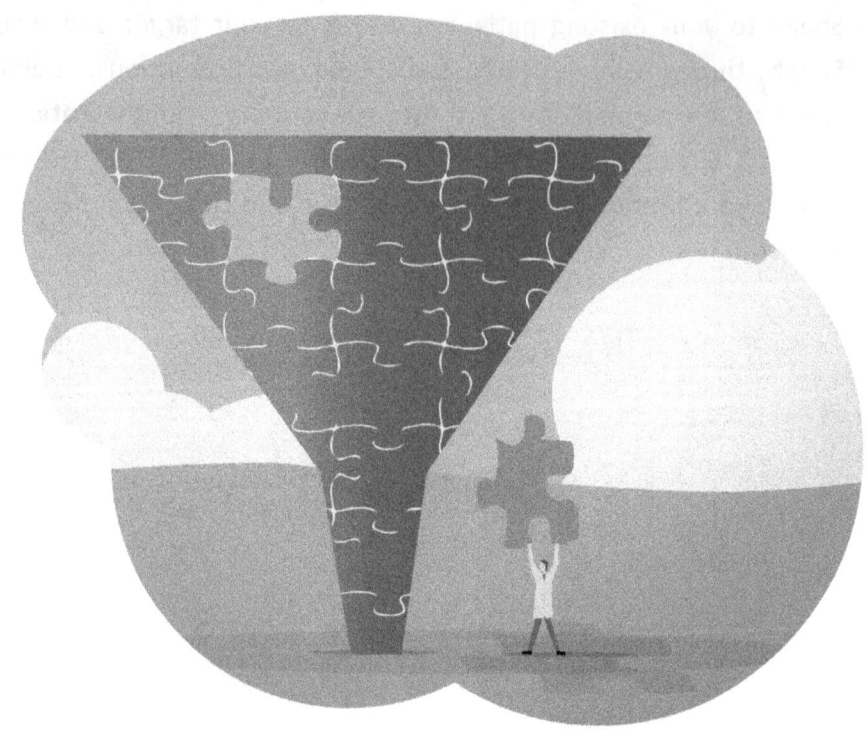

Putting It In Practice

There are so many businesses that put the cart (marketing communications) before the horse (branding). In fact, many don't ever get a horse, or even know what the horse if capable of doing. And if you can imagine how fruitless and exhausting it would be to pull a cart without a horse, you can see what it's like to spend time and money on brand-less marketing.

Up to this point, we've sold you the horse, giving you a fundamental appreciation for the (horse-?) power of branding. And now we get to show you how to put it to work through your marketing plan.

But first things first...your horse needs a name.

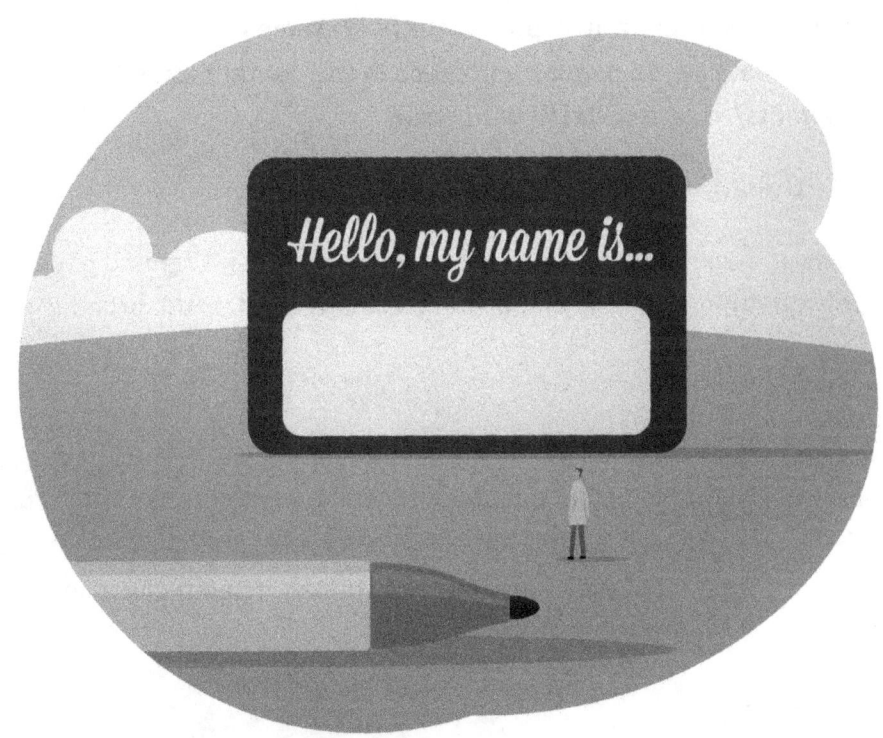

Choosing A Brand Name

You may be an established dental practice with a well-known and respected name; and if that's the case, then you can disregard this section. If you are a new practice, or a growing practice with new partners, or you are shifting the focus or specialization of your practice, then we're calling your name, so to speak...

Selecting a brand name can be a tricky decision. In the dental world, practice names are, more often than not, either the name of the practitioner (Phil Young, DDS) or affiliated with a geographic place (Dentistry of Charlotte or Cedar Lake Dentists). And while both choices are logical and valid, there are other options to be considered before you put Chiwetel Ejiofor, DDS (good thing he's an actor, not a dentist) or Bay Area Dentistry (B.A.D.) on the wall.

In general, there are 4 approaches (with some potential combinations) to naming a practice in the dental profession, and benefits/risks associated with each:

1. Using The Dentist's Name

If your own name is easy to pronounce and doesn't remind patients of something painful, you might consider using it as the brand.

Benefits:

- You, as the dentist, get immediate recognition
- In medicine, people often trust people before they trust generic organizations; personalizing the brand with the dentist's name sometimes makes it seem friendlier and more accessible

Risks:

- Names, and sometimes illogical patient biases against them, can be difficult
- If your name is on the door, patients expect to see you – any associate will automatically be considered inferior; and if you intend to add associates down the road, they will probably want their names in lights too
- If your 30-year plan is to eventually sell your business (and you don't have a buyer/benefactor with the same last name), your strong brand recognition will become a weakness for someone who wants to purchase and make it his/her own

2. Using a Geographic Designation

Benefits

- Brand names based on location are easy to pronounce, recognize and remember
- Town names or familiar geographic locations give a practice a hometown/neighborhood feel, creating immediate comfort and affiliation
- If the location conjures up the right imagery and associations, geography can be a big bonus (e.g. Lake Placid Dentistry)

Risks

- If you plan on expanding into other regions, the name may create confusion or negative associations (e.g. Los Angeles Dentistry might not be well-received in the Bay Area of San Francisco)
- If the name is based on obscure geography (e.g. a street name) it won't be memorable; if it's too broad (Dallas Dentistry), there might be several other practices with the location in the name (Dentistry of Dallas, Dallas Dental Group, etc.) that could create confusion.

Contriving a Name

Many medical practices create names that are either generic (ProCare Dentistry), symbolic (Sunny Day Dental) or benefit-based (SmileBright Dentistry).

Benefits

- Contrived names can create immediate connotations for the kind of care you offer and/or the way the patient will feel before, during and after the care
- If it's descriptive, yet unique, there is little risk of confusion or competitive issues

Risks

- In medicine, if a name is too cute or clever, the practice won't be taken seriously
- If too generic, a name loses its punch and memorability

Using Descriptors

Many practices use what are called 'descriptors' in branding. These include words such as: Family, Advanced, Pediatric, Professional, 24-Hour, Cosmetic, or Expert.

Benefits:

- Descriptors describe, so it's a good way to convey a specialization to attract the appropriate patients
- It allows you to clearly communicate your positioning (e.g. Expert Dentistry of Shaker Heights) to differentiate you from your competitors

Risks:

- Descriptors sometimes just add clutter to an already cumbersome name – make sure they are targeted and impactful
- If you begin as a niche dentist (e.g. pediatric) and want to grow your scope of expertise, you may have to "rebrand" later to broaden the name

In general, these are the 5 characteristics of a good name:

1. Pronounceable
2. Relatable
3. Memorable
4. Extendible
5. Distinctive

Also, remember that you have to be able to trademark and protect your name, so make sure that you do your homework on trademark availability and registration.

Go to www.uspto.gov for more information.

You could hire a branding company that specializes in name development (there are many and fees vary widely). However, if you are clear about what you want your brand to communicate, you should be able to develop a name on your own that captures that message and stays true to your personality.

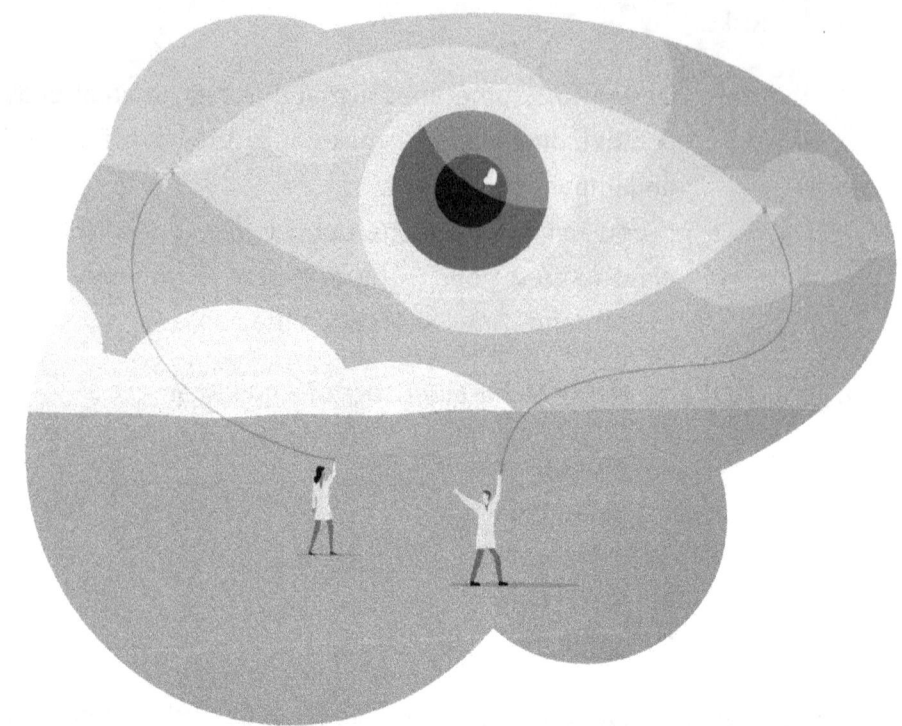

Crafting The Visual Brand Experience

Seeing is believing. So much of what we learn in the world is from seeing. And much of the time we don't realize the impact that colors, shapes, space, aesthetics, etc. have on us. That's why bringing a brand to life, visually, is as important as talking about it.

Creating A Logo & Color Scheme

After deciding on a name, many businesses get all excited about designing a fun, colorful logo without any thought as to how that logo needs to symbolize the brand. Your logo is a key tool in communicating your positioning. If you are a high-tech endodontist and your logo is of a cartoon mouth, you immediately confuse your message. Conversely, if you are a pediatric dentist and you choose black, silver and brown as your color scheme, you're missing the mark as well by not appealing to children.

Logos can incorporate symbols or icons (like Apple's apple or Target's bulls-eye) or they can just be font-based (like Google or Crest toothpaste). Many medical practices opt not to use an icon. However, even if you decide not to create a separate symbol, you need to be very deliberate about the font and color scheme that you use to represent your name. Every time you have a sign or a business card printed, the color & font need to be exactly the same.

If you look around at various healthcare-related businesses, you'll probably notice a lot of blue and green. That's because those colors are thought to represent nature, health, growth and professionalism. Blue, the color of sky and water, is also associated with purity, tranquility and stability. Green relates to the environment, "going", hope and luck. They are mostly positive messages to send out to people with health concerns.

Other colors can have conflicting messages, so designers are careful in how they use them. Yellow is cheerful and optimistic, but can also mean caution. Red can symbolize love and passion, but it is also the color of blood, debt and danger. Orange is warm and energetic, but it is seen as bold and flamboyant.

So you see how colors can have an impact, whether they are on your logo, your lettering, your walls or your website. You need to consider your practice type, your target audience and your brand positioning. Choose your color scheme carefully, and then be consistent in how you apply it, so that your audience begins to associate those colors with you and vice versa. Keep your logo files in one place on the computer so that staff can access it. Keep a list of rules (sometimes called an Identity Standards Manual) handy so that everyone is aware of exactly how the logo should be applied.

When designing a logo, you also need to consider how and where you will use it. It absolutely needs to look good on a sign, on your website and on a business card. But think beyond those essentials. Will you need to print it on scrubs? Pens? T-shirts? Toothbrushes?

As with a brand name, there are plenty of creative people out there that would love to develop a logo for you. And again, fees can vary widely (your friend, Joe, might sketch something for 50 bucks, and then there are the rumors that FedEx paid $1million to change their logo from FederalExpress to FedEx). Be sure that, if and when you hire someone, you are ready to articulate your brand vision and explain to him/her what you want that logo to say and represent. See if the designer is savvy about branding and "gets it" when you tell him that the logo needs to communicate your brand message.

If you think you might hire an artsy neighbor or an employee's cousin to design your logo, please reconsider. Your logo is critically important and, unless he or she is a professional graphic designer, you will probably regret the decision.

There are several design websites out there that are a great resource if you are on a budget. You provide a creative brief and determine the "prize" amount you'll pay for the winning design (as little as $150). Then thousands of designers around world decide if they want to submit designs for you and you typically end up with 50-100 designs from which to choose. Do an internet search for "logo design". You'd be surprised what you can get for $100.

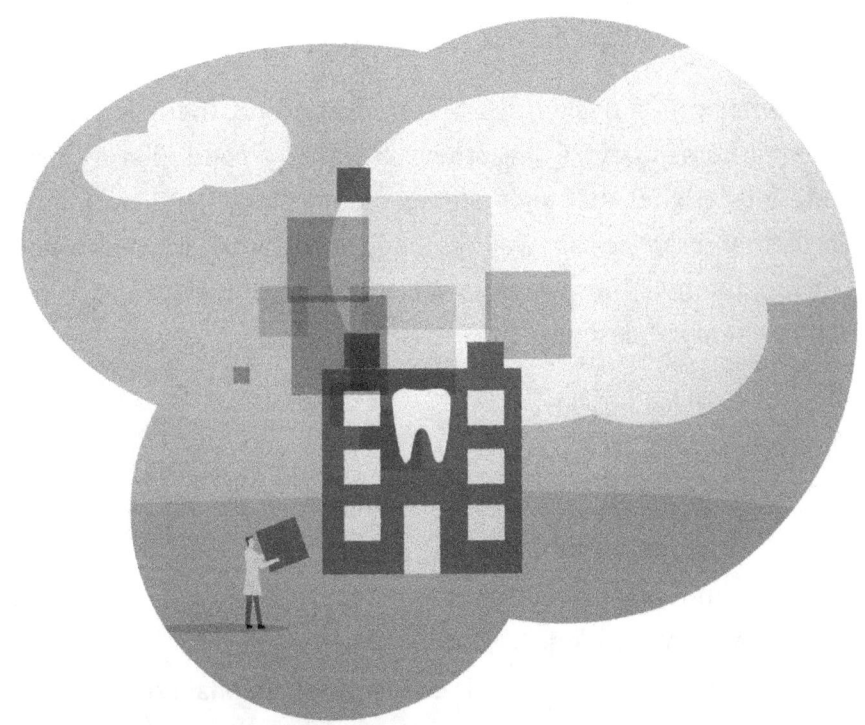

Designing The Office Experience

We talked earlier about customer "touch-points" and how every interaction with patients is an opportunity to let them see, touch and feel the brand. Office design is your first chance to validate your brand and create a positive, indelible image of who you are in your patients' minds. Stained carpets and dead fish in the tank immediately break your brand promise unless your practice name is "Dental Mediocrity".

Signage

As important as creating a compelling logo is putting that logo in prominent and effective places inside and outside your office. Make sure the sign is clear, professional and clean. How will they believe you can keep plaque off of their teeth if you can't keep dirt off your plaque?

Environmental Design

In dental office design, there is function and there is form and neither comes before the other. It's a very good idea to hire an interior designer that understands the mechanics and work-flow of a dental practice as well as the importance of the branded environment. Any customer-facing office should consider these components of design:

- Welcoming entry
- Clear way-finding
- Appropriate and consistent color scheme
- Appropriate furniture and decor
- Comfortable and tranquil waiting area
- Minimal work distraction
- Representation of staff culture and personality
- Accommodation of personal work styles
- Best use of lighting and temperature control
- Ability to adapt space to changing technology
- Ergonomics for both staff and patients
- Professionally-maintained plants (and perhaps, fish tank)

The greatest mistake business-owners make is to design solely based on their personal decorating tastes and styles. Now, we're sure you have lovely tastes, and of course you need to be comfortable with the design, but your target customers' needs and your brand personality should be the greater determining factors for the look and feel of the space. As with your logo, we highly recommend hiring a professional designer.

From your logo to your signs to your couches to your equipment, everything touches your patients in one way or another and if it impacts your patient, it impacts your brand.

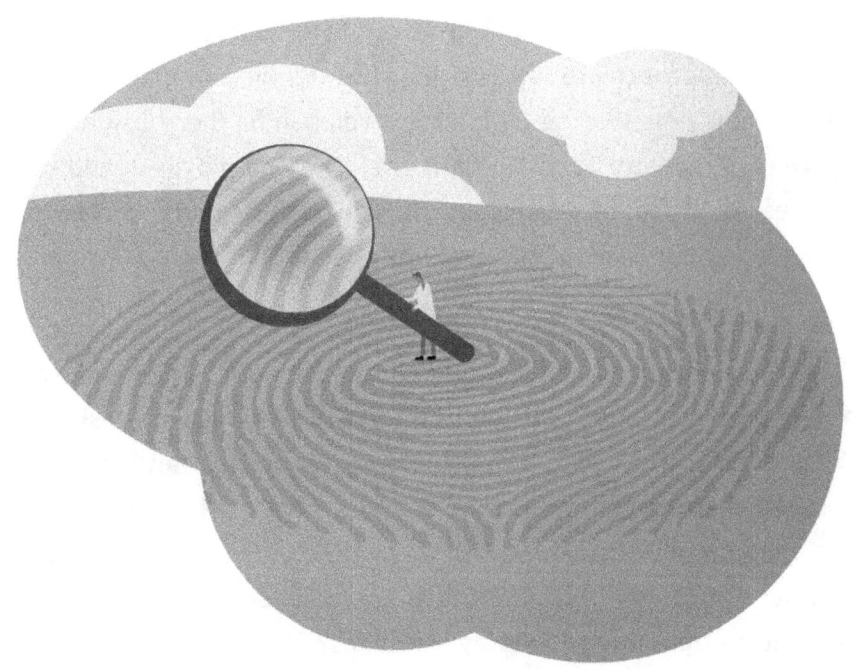

Creating The Personal Brand Experience

We've just told you how to approach the inanimate objects that affect your brand. Now let's move on to the animate ones (and we're not talking about the fish). People are a business' greatest asset. Period. And we're talking about both customers and staff. So how do we capitalize on those assets and best employ them to help grow our brands? Let's look at our staff first.

Employee Engagement

There's a reason they call it 'Human Resources': because humans are your greatest resource – particularly when it comes to growing your brand and your business. Once you arrive at your brand positioning, you need to "position" your staff to build that brand. Some call them ambassadors. Some call them advocates. We call them happy, engaged, empowered and proud employees.

Remember Richard Branson? The key to his success is his family-oriented approach to structuring the Virgin companies. Each employee is empowered by having a voice in his/her business and showing creativity and initiative. The employees and the businesses share ideas, values, interests and goals. They are engaged. They are collaborative. And they thrive.

You, or your office manager, probably spend hours training staff on the operations of your office and telling them where things are and how things are done. **But do you tell them about your vision for the practice? Do you tell them what your brand stands for? Do you tell them that they are an integral part of the organization and that brand?** Do you tell them to be creative about how they improve processes? Do you tell them to listen to customers and respond to their needs, whatever it takes? And after you tell them all of this, do you set aside time then, and in the future, to listen to their feedback, observations and ideas? You need to be doing all of that...and much more. You need to be engaging your staff.

You are all on the front line of your practice as far as your brand is concerned. Your office manager advocates the brand through marketing, employee training and operations. Your receptionist advocates the brand every time he or she greets a patient or answers the phone. Your hygienist advocates the brand through her conversation with the patient. And you, as the dentist, need to proactively advocate as well. You may be the most educated, most experienced dentist in town, but if your conversation and actions contradict your intended brand image, that's what the patient will remember...and he probably won't remember to come back.

Loyalty breeds loyalty. Respect breeds respect. Listening breeds ideas. Invest in training your employees. Solicit and invest in their insight. The more you listen to and value your employees' ideas, the more invested they will become in making your practice the best it can be. And your brand will thrive.

And while we're on the subject of staff, have you ever had an employee that was negatively affecting other staff and impacting the office harmony? Here's an idea on how to remove that person so you can get back to business.

Pay them to leave. While that sounds crazy at first, think about it. That disruptive person probably doesn't want to be there any more than you want them there. Offer them 1 month salary to leave and give them two days to make up their mind. Most likely, an unhappy employee will take the money and run and you just saved yourself 10 years of misery. Happy employees are a very important (and often overlooked) aspect of your brand.

Now let's examine the patient experience more closely and uncover how to increase engagement. A good friend and mentor Rolando Mia shared some insight many years ago that's been adapted to fit a dental practice. It's so simple, yet it's really the essence of this entire book – and we've made it into a simple tear out poster on the next page.

See what it is on the next page.

GET TO KNOW YOUR PATIENTS SO WELL,

YOU DON'T HAVE TO SELL

(Tear this page out and stick it to the bulletin board in the break room.

Read it every single day.)

Engaging the Patient

We've talked a lot about the individual elements that contribute to a brand experience in the practice. But now it's time to put it all together to see how it comes to life. It's called the 'Patient Experience'.

We mentioned earlier that you (or your staff) should walk in the patient's shoes to help craft your brand. We suggested visiting other practices and experiencing them with a critical eye. This lets you see what your competitors are doing well and not so well. You can then apply that insight and awareness to your business.

But you should also visit your own office with the perspective of a new patient. And/or recruit a few "trial customers" (staff, friends, family, neighbors) to be patients and report back to you. Take a critical look at the entryway and signage. What is your first impression when you walk through the door? How are you greeted? What is the lobby and check-in experience like? How was the cleaning and check-up process? How did the music, lighting, décor, temperature, office organization, background noises, etc. make you feel? Was the hygienist a Chatty Cathy, Moody Mary or Gentle Jane? How was the dentist's chair-side manner? What was missing (or should be missing, as the case may be) from the experience?

When you have these questions answered, see if those answers fit in with your intended brand position. Is it credible based on what you've seen and felt? Make changes based on the answers.

And then, when your practice is running the way the way you think it should be, ask your real patients. We talked earlier about surveys and having conversations about patient experiences to find out what needs are and aren't being met. You don't need to grill everyone who sits in the chair, but make a goal of talking to one or two a day, or a week, to find out how you can improve the experience and how you can tweak it to strengthen your brand.

As with your staff, by asking patients for feedback, you engage them in your brand. They feel valued and empowered and will, in turn, be more loyal to you and your practice brand. If you listen to them, they will listen to you...and your treatment recommendations.

Your communications skills are often the difference between a YES and a maybe, let's wait and see.

Stories are always more interesting than explanations. Become a better storyteller and make your treatment plan conversations more interesting and watch patient engagement and case acceptance increase.

Say it again –

Get to know your patients so well, you don't have to sell.

EXERCISE - #4 – DEFINE PATIENT EXPERIENCE

You've absorbed a lot about the patient experience. Now try to articulate your ideal patient experience in writing. Choose 2 ideal patients with different demographic profiles (e.g. a mother of 2 in her 30s and an empty-nester in his 50s). For each, describe: the patient, how he hears about you, what happens when she contacts you, when he walks in the lobby, when she meets the staff, when he sits in the chair, when she undergoes a procedure, when he checks out, when she is contacted again, etc. etc. Try to be as creatively descriptive as possible. Think outside the box. Big picture. Reach for the stars. And then decide which stars are most important, even if they seem unattainable right now.

The Ideal Patient Experience: _____

_____

_____

_____

_____

_____

_____

_____

_____

_____

_____

_____

_____

_____

_____

_____

_____

_____

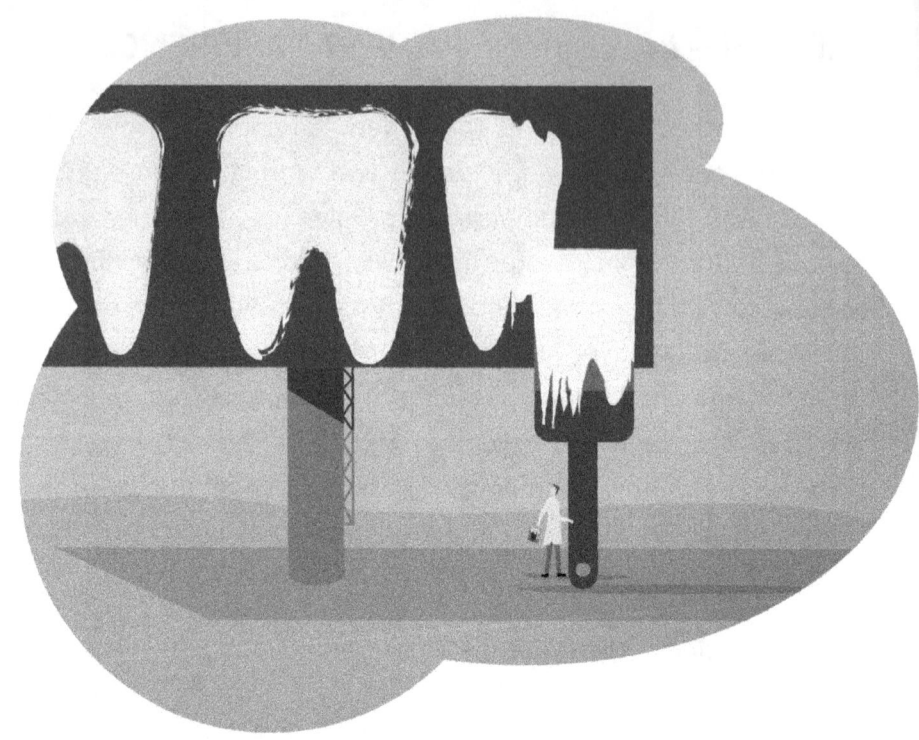

Creating The Public Brand Experience

The personal brand that we just discussed focuses on existing (both new and long term) patients – those that are definitely coming through the door and experiencing your practice. **Now we're going to add in the rest of your audience** – those that you want to come through your door, but haven't yet decided to. Your public brand is what everyone sees and hears, patients or not. It's how you're viewed in the greater community - on billboards, in newspapers, on TV and online. It's how you're talked about – through word of mouth, in the press, and on Facebook. It's called 'Marketing Communications' and it involves every communication your practice, and your brand, makes with the outside world. Turn the page and let's see what kind of marketing is right for you.

The Components of Marketing Communications

A. Offline (or Traditional) Marketing

When most people without a marketing degree think of marketing, they often think of advertising. While they are not synonymous, advertising is a critical component of building any strong product or service brand. Here is a run-down of TRADITIONAL advertising and promotion options you might consider to help build your brand:

- **Radio** – Radio advertising can be effective if it is kept simple since you can never be sure that you have listeners' full attention. MP3 players and satellite radio have diluted the potency of AM/FM radio as well. There are so many terrible radio ads out there, as it's difficult to create something catchy yet professional with only sounds and no visuals. But if you can find just the right creative radio ad concept and execution, great. If not, you might consider sponsorship of traffic reports or news updates...or redirecting your advertising funds to another medium. **The trick here is making sure your target market you defined earlier is listening here**.

- **Television** – It's expensive and relatively untrackable as far as its effectiveness goes - particularly for a small, usually local, business like a dental practice. Big brands use it and use it well, but without a solid creative budget and some left over for great ad placement and repetition, it can be a waste of money and effort for dentists. An exception might be an infomercial of a very specific topic/niche – like migraine treatment or pain free dentistry.

- **Print** (newspaper, magazines, etc.) – Because print is familiar and relatively easy to execute, it remains popular for small businesses. Its effectiveness can be difficult to track, but it can be successful if you take the time to find just the right targeted publications and you are consistent in your brand message.

- **Outdoor** (billboards, transit media - bus benches/shelters, automobile & building wraps, street signage, etc.) – Location. Location. Location. Outdoor advertising can be extremely effective and useful depending on the nature and location of your practice. Billboards and street signs are great for local awareness and leading them directly to your location. Transit media is often affordable and you have a captive audience willing and able to read the message.

- **Direct Mail** – Most small, local, service businesses can (and should) use direct mail effectively. If you have a well-maintained database and you purchase the right lists that allow you to target through demographics (like geography, age, family status, spending habits, etc.), it can be a beneficial way to promote your practice. Google does direct mail – enough said.

- **Flyers/Brochures** – Also easy to create, but relatively expensive to produce, flyers and pamphlets should be distributed (or available for grabbing) only in targeted locations. Standing on a random street corner and handing them to every passerby is not a good use of funds. But posting flyers or placing brochures in daycare centers or school offices might be a good approach for a pediatric dentist. But be sure they'll let you leave them before you print them!

- **Community Involvement & Sponsorship** – Local businesses, such as dentists, need to be locally involved. Whether you are giving an annual speech on the importance of dental health at a local high school or sponsoring a little league team or charitable event, you need to connect with, and participate in your community.   It creates visibility and awareness and it allows you to project your brand on a more personal level.

- **Interdisciplinary Marketing** – Unique to certain businesses and professions (like dentistry) is the use of interdisciplinary marketing – marketing to and through other professionals. You should be marketing yourself to physicians and other healthcare providers. If you are a specialist such as an endodontist, you should be marketing yourself to general practitioners. And make it go both ways. Referrals are like boomerangs – throw one out there and one usually comes back to you.

STATISTIC ALERT

13% of people trust advertising

70% trust people they DON'T know

90% trust people they DO know

B. Online (or Internet) Marketing

Like it or not, we are in the digital age. So, no matter how compelling your radio ads, or how targeted your direct mail, you will not beat your competitors or maximize your practice without an online marketing strategy. Below is a list of online marketing tools that you should be implementing:

- **Website Design** – Your website is as important as your lobby these days (many might say WAY more important). Think about it, a patient will never see your your lobby without seeing your website first. It's most likely the first impression patients get of your practice. It needs to be clean, professional, easy to navigate and in line with your brand position. There are thousands of website development companies out there. But be wary. We highly recommend hiring someone that is multi-disciplined in their approach - knowing design, branding, online marketing SEO and SEM.

- **SEO (Search Engine Optimization)** – SEO creates greater visibility and a higher ranking of your website in a search engine's innate or "unpaid" search results. It optimizes website content, keywords, links and HTML code to promote your site and create greater traffic.

- **Reputation Management** – Reputation management is extremely important. From making sure your local listings are current and accurate (so you get found) to getting reviews on Google, Yelp and Facebook . This is definitely something to outsource to someone who can stay on this 24/7. **It's that important.**

- **SEM (Search Engine Marketing)** – This is a form of online advertising used to increase awareness through "paid" placements on specific sites, contextual advertising and paid inclusion on search engine sites like Google, Yahoo and Bing. Some people call this Google AdWords, but that only gets you on Google which accounts for about 2/3rds of search volume. That means if you only use Google AdWords, you are missing 1 out of every 3 people who are searching the web for your services. A good SEM strategy involves ALL search engines. You should probably hire a professional for this service.

- **Email** – Email can be a great tool for marketing through newsletters, educational information, appointment reminders and loyalty programs. Although it is incredibly more cost-effective than direct mail, it is more sensitive as far as privacy and spam concerns go. Even if patients opt-in to receiving emails, be efficient and effective in your communication. Less is more if you do it right. Again, ensure that your email design and language is consistent with your brand messaging and other marketing materials.

- **Blogs** – Businesses that blog statistically get over 50% more traffic than those that don't. If it's interesting and relevant to your audience, write about it, post it, and make it easy for people to share it and pass it along. Show people how informed, experienced and insightful you are. If people start listening to your blog, they'll start listening to your treatment suggestions too. Have your staff write. There are countless sources of information to post to a blog. And countless benefits to doing so. Just make sure to blog on a regular basis – frequency and consistency are important.

- **Social Media** - Although originally designed for personal interaction, social media has become essential for businesses. You should have accounts with Facebook, Twitter, Linkedin, YouTube, and Google+, to name a few. They keep you on the radar of your audience. They let you create a sense of community with your business. And they have vast reach through networks, enabling you to promote your business well beyond the scope of any email or direct mail campaign. Facebook and Twitter can get you innumerable endorsements. A YouTube channel lets you post and share a video of your practice or the latest and greatest technology that you're using. If you're not using social media, you're old school. If you're old school, you're not innovating. And these days, if you're not innovating, your business is going backwards.

- **Online Promotions / Coupons** – Groupon, Living Social, AmazonLocal, Angie's List...the list of online promotion sites grows daily. They have been good instruments for getting a bump in business. Who wouldn't think $49 for a check-up, cleaning, x-rays and teeth whitening system is a great deal? And we are not going to tell you not to use them. However, there are a few pitfalls to consider. First, there are a lot of them out there now, so deals don't seem quite as special or compelling anymore; but you don't want to make them SO compelling that you lose money. Second, there are a lot of people that coupon-hop, i.e. they go for the one cleaning with one dentist and then wait for another coupon 6 months later and start over with another dentist. And lastly, if you provide them too often, you end up devaluing your services. Online coupons can be a good way to boost awareness every so often, but don't count on coupon users translating into long-term, loyal paying patients.

Determining Marketing Communications Strategy

All dentists **MUST** have a marketing communications plan, but there are several questions to answer before you decide if this is something you and your team can handle internally, or if it is something you should outsource to a trusted partner.

1. **What is my budget?**

    You will need to be very thoughtful in your advertising strategy, and creative in your tactical approach. Consider all of your options and know the numbers - i.e. what is the viewership (TV), circulation (print), traffic/clicks (internet.

    And remember, it's not just the media type that costs money; you will have to pay creative costs as well.

2. **Who am I targeting?**

    If you are a general dentist, your target is wide and many forms of media will be relevant to your marketing communications strategy. You might buy billboard space, as the reach is more general. If you are a pediatric dentist, you are probably targeting the moms that make 90% of their family's healthcare decisions. Your money might be better spent on more specific media, such as local parenting magazines and websites.

3. **What is my message and how is it building my brand?**

    Everyone likes to have their name in lights for all the world to see. And advertising and promotion does just that. But ironically, just when businesses have the opportunity to reach their target audience, they make one of 2 mistakes:

- They go 'creative crazy' and try to make something splashy, clever, artsy or silly that either neglects to communicate their brand message or, worse, contradicts it. Your ads, brochures, website, etc. should be eye-catching, but they must also be consistent with, and work to build, your brand.
- They go 'home-made'. Marketing on a budget is an art in and of itself. But having your receptionist create your magazine ad, or your neighbor develop your website, is a bad idea unless he or she has expertise in the area. You must be professional in all of your communications.

4. Can my internal team handle this?

Marketing is serious business. Just like your taxes and your financial planning. Marketing requires expertise, a solid plan and execution.

On the next page, we talk about the very first step every practice should take BEFORE starting any marketing campaign. This simple process can save thousands of dollars and more importantly time.

Reputation & Review Marketing

Warren Buffet famously said *'It takes 20 years to build a reputation and five minutes to ruin it. If you think about that, you'll do things differently.'* And with our 24/7 culture and the speed of the Internet, those words couldn't be more true today. Your reputation is very, very important. To survive and thrive, you must develop it, protect it and market it. It's an extension of you and it's a big part of your brand.

An easy way to manage your reputation is through online reviews and feedback. Online reviews are all around us. When you book a hotel or choose a restaurant, most likely you depend on a review to help you make your decision. Your patients are no different. Patients read reviews, patients write reviews, patients trust reviews. Positive reviews are the cornerstone of building your reputation online.

There are several companies that can help you – you can do an online search for 'Reputation Marketing for Dentists' to see a list. One company that I've worked with (in a partnership with one of my clients) is BirdEye. They are focused in dentistry and have the robust software to help guide you through this process. Here is what they do -

- Competitive analysis and report
- Identify inconsistencies in your local listings
- Help get you found on Google and other search engines
- Get positive reviews directly on Google, Yelp and Facebook
- Monitor and protect your reputation

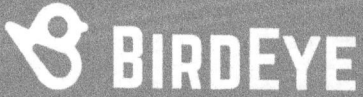

Learn more
www.brandtarget.com/reputation
Use code BRAND for no setup fee

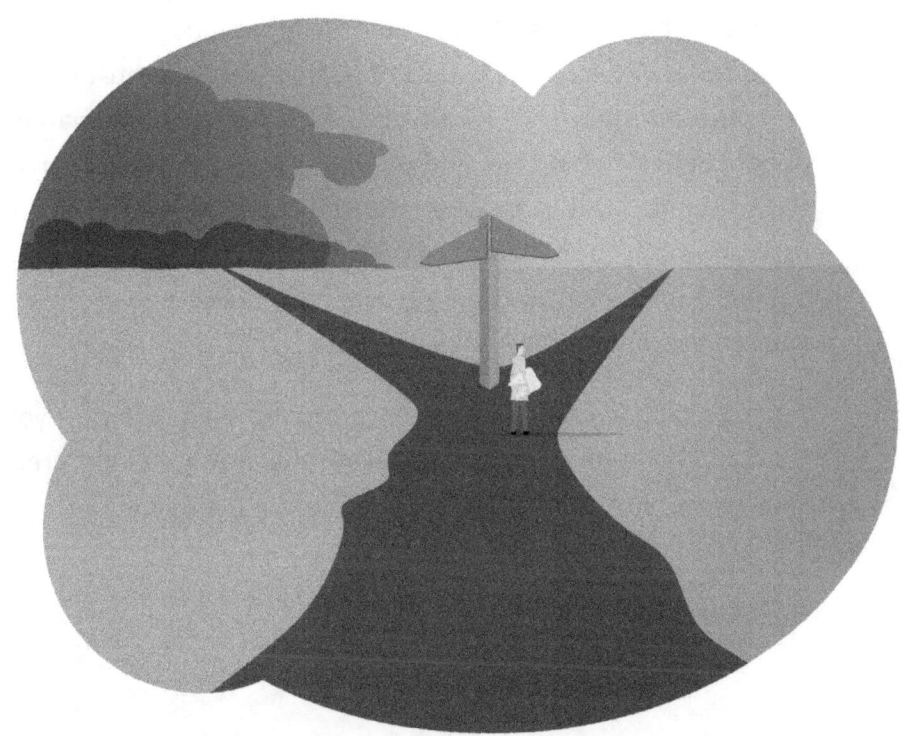

Walk The Talk Of Marketing

Like it or not, people have become more skeptical in the world. Some blame it on the media. Some blame politicians. Some blame consumerism and the elusive promise of greatness. Advertisers have bought a lot of air time and sold a lot of air over the years and we're not sure which claims of greatness to believe anymore. The phrase "Trust me" often means "You really shouldn't."

It's why reviews from places like Yelp, Angie's List and Google have become so important. A few years ago, if a person moved to a new town and wanted to find a new dentist, they probably picked the one closest to their house that is also covered by their insurance plan. This was how we all did it, mostly because we didn't have access to the kind of information that is out there today. These days, you can't be an average dentist with a un-educated staff giving bad customer service. **Ultimately, people believe what they find on their own – not what's force-fed to them.** Make sure what you say about yourself matches up with what your patients are saying about you. Make sure the patient experience matches up with the brand. Make sure your online reputation is squeaky clean.

You can talk the talk (advertise, promote, blog, etc.) all you want, but only those that truly walk the walk (provide great care and service) win and keep customers in the end.

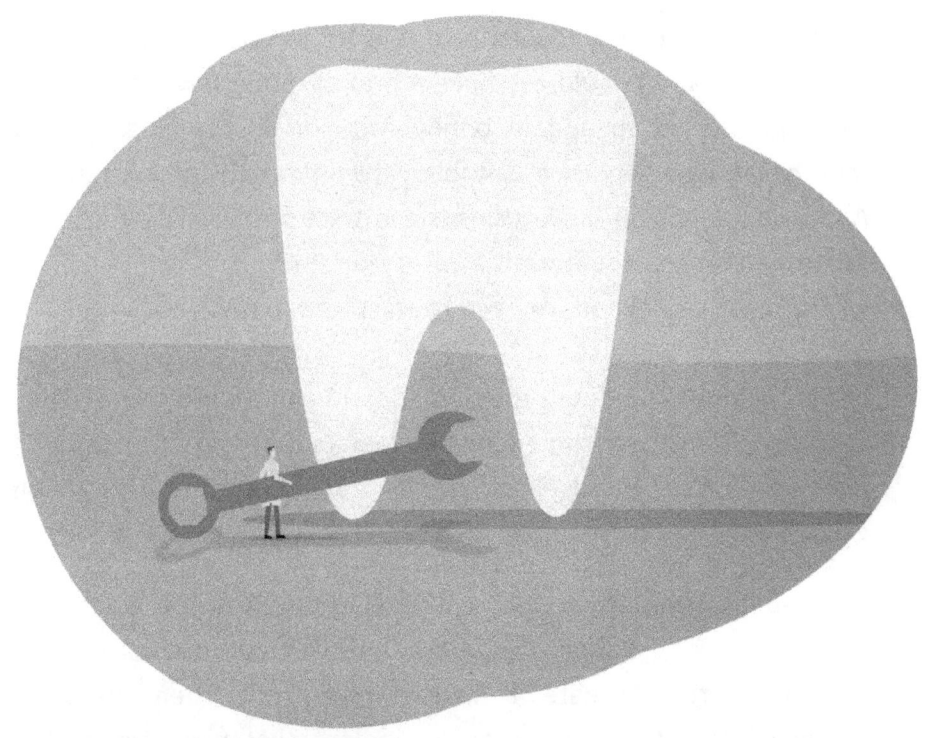

The Brand Check-Up

MONITORING & MOTIVATING YOUR BRAND

You know how, after patients go to the dentist, they start flossing daily, they brush for twice as long, perhaps even after every meal. Then, a few weeks later, they floss every other day, brushing only twice a day. Then, a few months later, flossing is a weekly event and brushing is on auto-pilot, giving their teeth a few strokes running out the door. But then comes the 6-month check-up/cleaning and the whole process is rebooted and re-energized, and the daily flossing happens again. Without that 6-month check-up, they might even stop flossing altogether.

Well, branding and marketing undergo a similar process. When we first create our brand, we come up with a clever campaign, we get excited about it, we advertise in every medium, we blog every hour, and lo and behold, we have a brand! But a few weeks later, we might forget to update our website or post a blog. A few months later we get lazy about following up on satisfaction surveys. And a year later, our advertising is spotty at best, our posters have faded and so has the enthusiasm of our staff. We find ourselves with a faded brand and we need to start from scratch once again.

Branding and marketing require discipline and a daily ritual. They require continual benchmarking to evaluate how the brand is doing and how it can improve and evolve. **So here's the 4-Rs to an effective marketing regime:**

> **Step 1: Regulate** – Once you decide on what you want your brand to be, you have to define the rules that are going to get you there.   Create a marketing plan.   Then create a weekly/monthly routine to implement that plan. Define the roles that each employee plays in making the whole "brand performance" come together.   Appoint a staff member to monitor the brand. This is really important. If someone is not ultimately accountable for following through on brand management, it will never happen.   If you didn't keep an appointment schedule, your practice would be a mess. If you don't keep a brand planner, your practice brand will be a mess.

> **Step 2: Review** - Once you decide to build a brand, commit to a 3- or 6-month check-up to make sure you're on track and where you want to be.   Analyze what's working and what's not. Compare patient satisfaction surveys and track your progress (or lack thereof). Keep talking to your staff, your patients, your wider target audience, and find out how they perceive your brand. Continue to monitor your competitors and the dental profession overall.

Step 3: Revise – After reviewing and comparing, identify the gaps and the new challenges facing the business and the brand. Revise your marketing plan to ensure that you close those gaps. You might increase your advertising budget or commit more resources to stepping up your social media presence. Analyze each aspect and see if it's working. If it's not, change it up.

Step 4: Refresh – Never let your brand stagnate. Even if you've done a good job in developing a cohesive and compelling brand over a few years, you need to refresh it so that it continues to shine and catch the eye of all patients – new, old and targeted. It might be as simple as a new coat of paint, new fish and a new way of greeting patients. Or you might shift your overall brand positioning in response to new competitors or adding disciplines to your own practice. "Just Do It" is considered one of the greatest taglines of all times, but even Nike refreshed its brand with a new tagline after several years.

You can't do an initial marketing campaign and expect it to work for years to come. It doesn't work that way. **Even the Super Bowl runs advertising to remind you to watch it.** Marketing is a never-ending process. Just when you think you're done, something changes. Maybe it's a new competitor in your zip code. Maybe it's a dip in the economy that slows your business down. Maybe it's a new technology that helps you connect with prospects. Whatever the change, you can only tread water for so long before you sink. In today's economy, you're either moving forward or getting passed by. You need to maintain and even gain momentum in your branding efforts if you are to be truly successful.

Just like life, branding is a journey, not a destination.

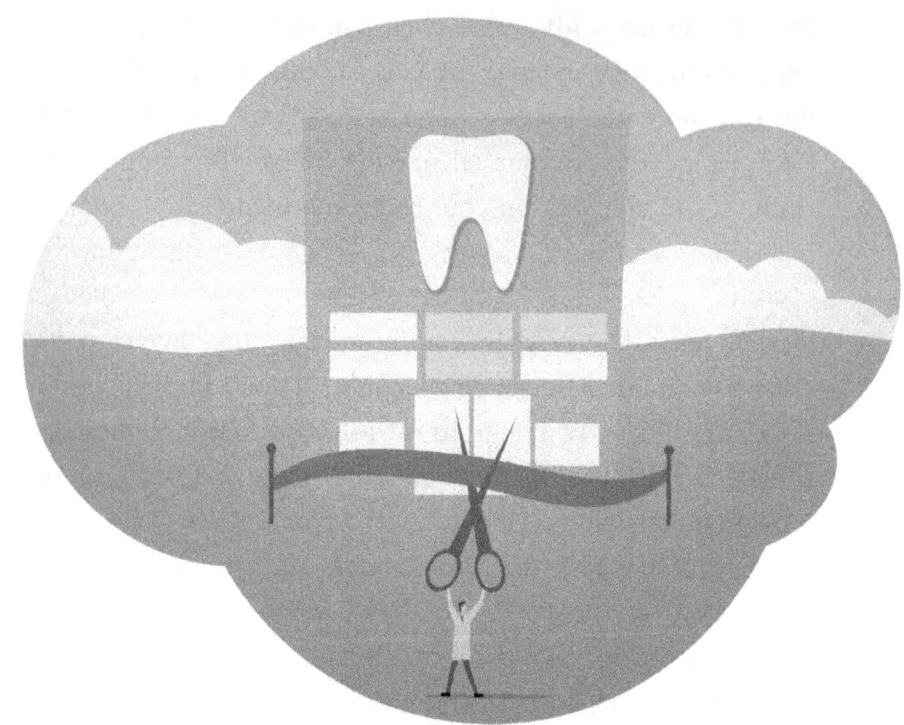

Let The Branding Begin

We have talked at length about many components and tactics of branding and marketing and how they all work together. But we want to be clear that branding can be as simple or complex as you make it. And often times the simple approach is the most effective.

Articulate where you want to be in 1 year, 5 years, 10 years and then make a plan to get there. Make sure that it is both aspirational and realistic. If you have budget constraints, choose efficient and inexpensive ways to develop and communicate your brand. Maybe you just talk to your patients for now instead of deploying an online survey. Maybe you only email, blog and redesign your website in the first year instead of investing in advertising. Or maybe you're ready, strategically and financially, to jump in with both feet and do it all.

The bottom line is: If you can be clear in what you want your brand to be, and be consistent in how you present it, your dental practice will win the branding game soon...and often.

So the branding journey begins. You define your target audience and you listen to it. Always. You determine your unique positioning and you own it. Always. You prove yourself, promote yourself and outdo yourself. Always and forever.

To help you start your journey, we've put together a quick list of what to do and what not to do:

DON'T: Procrastinate any longer on taking the first step in developing a 'consumer-centric' brand

DO: Set realistic goals of what you want your practice to look/feel like - TREAT YOUR PATIENTS LIKE CONSUMERS

DON'T: Underestimate the power of your patients' insight – they know more and can influence your business more than you think

DO: Create an ongoing conversation with existing patients and target customers – solicit feedback, ideas, 'intel' on competitors

DON'T: Hire a non-professional friend or family member to help you market your practice, design a logo or anything for that matter

DO: Hire professionals when you are out of your comfort zone (website, office design, etc.)

DON'T: Keep doing the same thing over and over and expect different results

DO: Continually re-evaluate everything that touches the customer (signage, receptionist, greeting, email, lobby/waiting area, uniform)

DON'T: Think that your dental expertise will speak for itself

DO: Share your expertise and brand personality with the world through blogs, YouTube videos and other communications

DON'T: Let newer, younger dentists brand themselves while you watch it happen

DO: Remember that stronger brands charge more and retain more customers

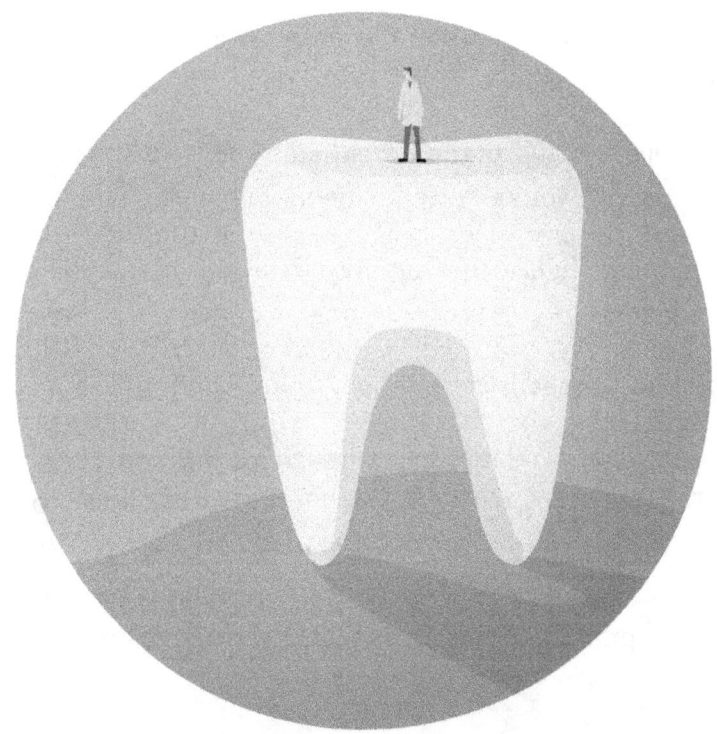

Conclusion

The world is vastly different today than it was just ten or fifteen years ago. As a small business owner, you have more tools and channels to reach your customers than ever before. This can seem intimidating, but in this competitive environment you must use this to your advantage. However, before the marketing begins, the brand has to be right from the start.

Connecting with your prospects and patients is more vital than ever. Consumers want to connect with the companies they buy from. Consumers want to connect with you. Once you make the shift in your mind to treat your practice like a consumer brand, everything changes. The focus shifts from just treating patient's teeth to treating consumers wants *and* needs.

Branding's logic is based on the simple principle that "if you build it, they will come".

If you build a brand that differentiates you from your competition and shows why you're better, patients will see it and value it.

If your brand fulfills that promise in every interaction, they will keep coming.

If your brand exceeds expectations, their friends will come too.

If you develop a relationship through your brand, they will trust you. The more they trust you, the more they will listen to you. The more they listen to you, the higher your case acceptance. And higher case acceptance leads to a happier you and a more successful practice. Whew, that's quite a progression.

Go ahead

Be   A

Brand

www.ingramcontent.com/pod-product-compliance
Lightning Source LLC
Chambersburg PA
CBHW051813170526
45167CB00005B/1993